>> **15** minute
everyday
pilates

Alycea Ungaro P.T.

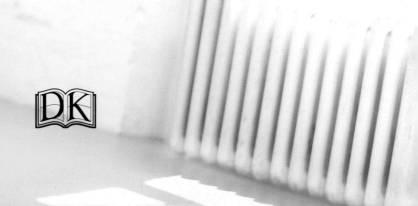

DK

London, New York, Melbourne, Munich and Delhi

For my husband Robert

Project Editor Hilary Mandleberg
Project Art Director Miranda Harvey
Senior Art Editor Peggy Sadler
Managing Editor Penny Warren
Managing Art Editor Marianne Markham
Art Director Peter Luff
Publishing Director Mary Clare Jorram
Stills Photography Ruth Jenkinson
DTP Designer Sonia Charbonnier
Production Controllers Rebecca Short, Sarah Sherlock
Production Editor Luca Frassinetti
Jacket Designer Neal Cobourne

DVD produced for Dorling Kindersley by
Chrome Productions www.chromeproductions.com

Director Joel Mishcon
DOP Marcus Domleo, Matthew Cooke
Camera Marcus Domleo, Jonathan Iles
Production Manager Hannah Chandler
Production Assistant Nathan Nikolov
Grip Pete Nash
Gaffer Paul Wilcox, Johann Cruickshank
Music Chad Hobson
Hair and Makeup Roisin Donaghy, Victoria Barnes
Voiceover Alycea Ungaro
Voiceover Recording Charles de Montebello, CDM Studios,
New York City (www.cdmstudios.com)

First published in Great Britain in 2008
by Dorling Kindersley Limited
80 Strand, London WC2R 0RL
Penguin Group (UK)

Health warning
All participants in fitness activities must assume the responsibility
for their own actions and safety. If you have any health problems
or medical conditions, consult with your doctor before
undertaking any of the activities set out in this book. The
information contained in this book cannot replace sound
judgement and good decision making, which can help reduce
risk of injury. See also page 11.

A CIP catalogue record is available from the British Library

ISBN 978-1-4053-2658-2

Printed and Bound in China

Discover more at
www.dk.com

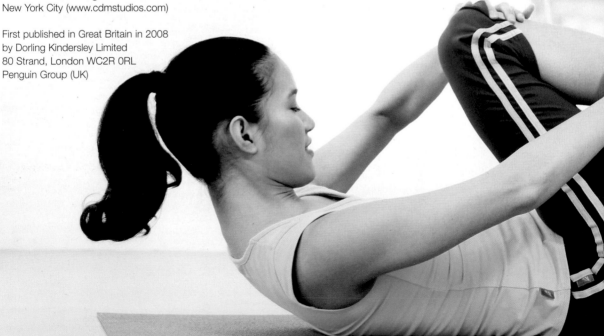

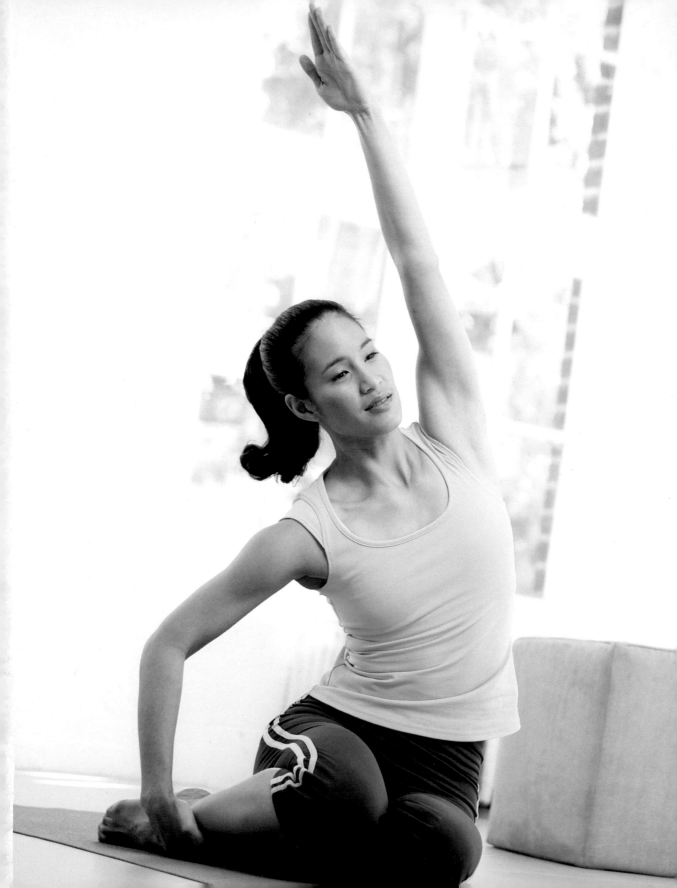

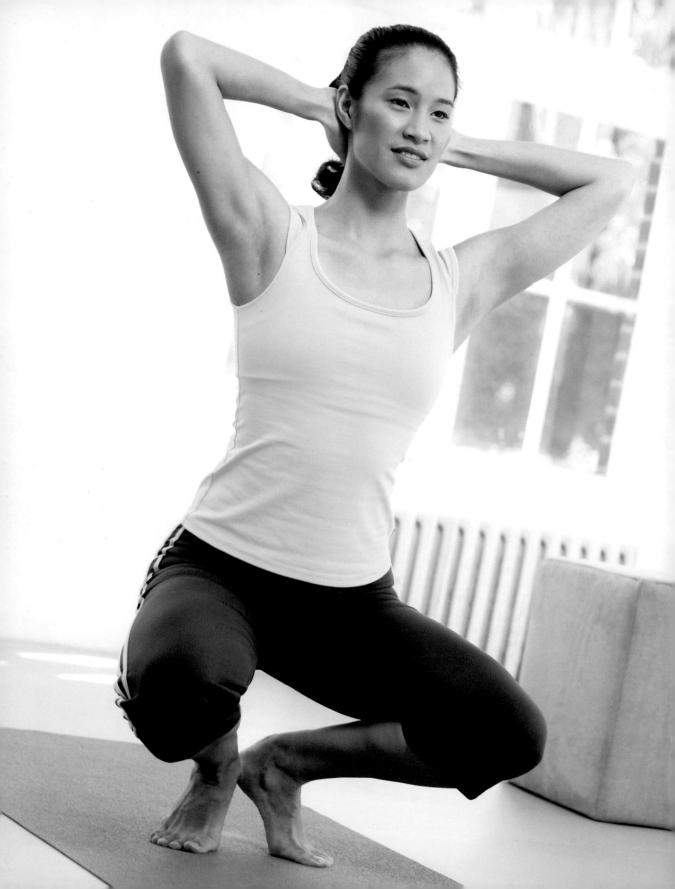

contents

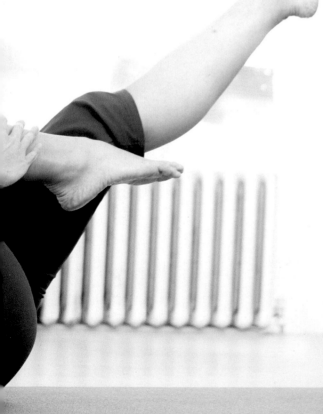

Author Foreword 6

sweatyBetty Foreword 7

How to Use this Book 8

Day by Day 18

Day by Day Summary 34

Day by Day Extras 40

From the Top Down 42

From the Top Down Summary 58

From the Top Down Extras 64

From the Bottom Up 66

From the Bottom Up Summary 82

From the Bottom Up Extras 88

Up, Up and Away 90

Up, Up and Away Summary 106

Up, Up and Away Extras 112

Beyond the Workout 114

Resources 124

Index 126

Acknowledgments 128

Health warning
Always consult your doctor before starting a fitness programme if you have any health concerns and especially if you are pregnant, have given birth in the last six weeks, or have a medical condition such as high blood pressure, arthritis, or asthma.

Every effort has been made to ensure that the information contained in this book is complete and accurate. However, neither the publisher nor the author is engaged in rendering professional advice or services to the individual reader. The ideas, information and suggestions contained in this book are not intended as a substitute for consulting with your physician. All matters regarding your health require medical supervision. Neither the author nor the publisher shall be liable or responsible for any loss or damage allegedly rising from any information or suggestion in this book.

>> **author** foreword

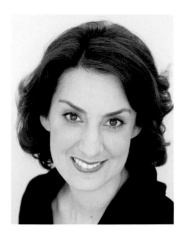

This collection of four Pilates programmes is meant as a tool, to teach, guide and inform and, hopefully, to inspire. The programmes will excite your body and mind into action and launch you into a lifetime of wellness and health.

Pilates is not 'just another workout'. Pilates goes where you do. It's a mindset, a perspective and a lifestyle. Approached in that way, Pilates guarantees results.

When I first signed on to this project, I was overwhelmed by the possibilities. Where to begin, I thought? Oddly, it was my practice of Pilates that gave me the wherewithal to accomplish the job. Pilates exercises are finite – or so I had been taught – in the same way as there has to be a finite number of words and images in this book. But the beauty of Pilates is that the more intimately you know the system, the more complex and fascinating it becomes. If you truly understand the method, you will always have the perfect exercise at your fingertips without having to beg, borrow or steal from any other method or technique. Everything you need is right there. By drawing on what I have learned over the 25 years I have been a student of Pilates, I have composed a novel approach to a brilliant and timeless method of exercise.

This project reignited my passion for Pilates in a whole new way. The constraints imposed upon me became utterly liberating. What a luxury once again to reinvent the familiar. Everyday Pilates is a new approach – one intended to drive home the mission of Pilates. That is, to get you living a better life – off the floor and out the door.

Here you have four distinct programmes that are derivative in nature. By and large, the choreography is pure Pilates. The order of exercises is my own and I believe the sequences to be effective and efficient, which is the hallmark of true Pilates work. Sadly, for the Pilates purist, there is no atlas to serve as a reliable resource for a concrete list of exercises. At best, we are piecing together memories that are subjective and interpretive. I so wish that Joe and Clara Pilates were here to share their gifts with us. I believe they would have been proud to see their work preserved yet progressing after all these years.

sweatyBetty foreword

I believe in healthy living, having fun, Cornish clotted cream and cool tracksuits!

Before I opened the first sweatyBetty boutique in London's trendy Notting Hill I had no major commitments. Outside of my 9 to 5 job my time was my own and keeping fit and healthy was fun and easy. Nowadays, with a husband, three kids and a whole chain of boutiques to look after, I have very little 'me' time!

I'm the first to admit that finding the time to work out can be a challenge but it's essential if, like me, you need to juggle your work and home life. So whilst I'm unlikely to run a marathon, swim the Channel or climb Everest in the near future, I can certainly do enough to keep myself looking and feeling good.

We can all find a spare 15 minutes, a few times a week, in the comfort of our own home to keep our bodies and minds in check. So I encourage you to get off the sofa and get active, in sweatyBetty gear of course…!

Tamara Hill-Norton

Founder of sweatyBetty
the UK's leading women's activewear retailer

>> **how to** use this book

Welcome to *Everyday Pilates.* These four 15-minute programmes are the closest you can get to having a personal trainer right by your side. They offer you the flexibility and ease of use that our busy lifestyles demand. *Everyday Pilates* is meant to accomplish your everyday goals for your everyday life!

I am a huge fan of clichés. One that comes to mind when considering how best to approach these programmes is, 'Be prepared, or be prepared to fail'. The biggest mistake you can make is to dive into the material without reading this book or watching the DVD. Pilates can be tricky. Exercises may appear to focus on one area but actually are intended to accomplish something different.

There are several tools to help you understand the details. The DVD is designed to be used with the book to reinforce the exercises shown there. As you watch the DVD, page references to the book flash up on the screen. Refer to these pages for more detailed instruction.

On each page, the photographs capture the essence of the exercises in simple step-by-step images. Some exercises require two or three images, while others only require one. Certain exercises contain smaller inset photos that depict the first step. You will also find targeted 'feel-it-here' graphics on specific exercises. These are intended to emphasize the fact that there is always a different area of the body to focus on.

The gatefolds

If I had a pound for every time a client asked me if we had a chart of the Pilates exercises – well, you can work out the rest! Luckily for you, at the end of each programme, a gatefold chart of the exercises follows. These are meant to provide at-a-glance reminders. You won't be able to learn how to do the exercises from the gatefolds since we have

pared down the images there, providing only one or two per exercise as your reminder. But once you have watched the DVD, read through the book and practised each move thoroughly, these gatefolds will become invaluable. For tips on how often to perform the programmes and how to combine them for longer workouts, see pp116–117.

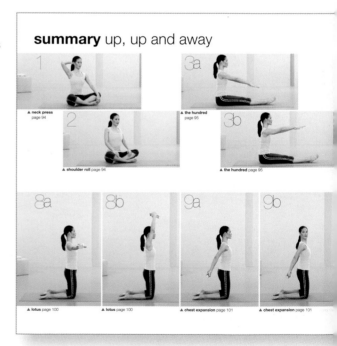

The gatefolds At-a-glance charts will help further your practice once you no longer need the step-by-step images. Review the full programme before beginning.

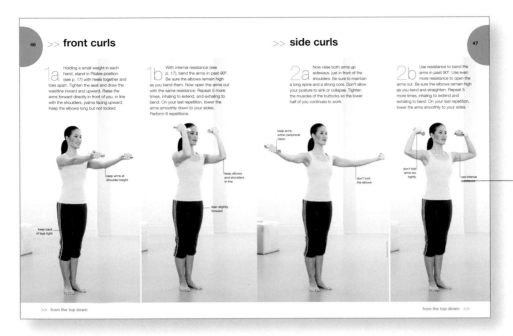

>> front curls

1a Holding a small weight in each hand, stand in Pilates position (see p. 17) with heels together and toes apart. Tighten the seat and draw the waistline inward and upward. Raise the arms forward directly in front of you, in line with the shoulders, palms facing upward. Keep the elbows long but not locked.

1b With internal resistance (see p. 17), bend the arms in past 90°. Be sure the elbows remain high as you bend them. Now open the arms out with the same resistance. Repeat 5 more times, inhaling to extend, and exhaling to bend. On your last repetition, lower the arms smoothly down to your sides. Perform 6 repetitions.

>> side curls

2a Now raise both arms up sideways, just in front of the shoulders. Be sure to maintain a long spine and a strong core. Don't allow your posture to sink or collapse. Tighten the muscles of the buttocks so the lower half of you continues to work.

2b Use resistance to bend the arms in past 90°. Use even more resistance to open the arms out. Be sure the elbows remain high as you bend and straighten. Repeat 5 more times, inhaling to extend and exhaling to bend. On your last repetition, lower the arms smoothly to your sides.

keep arms at shoulder-height

keep back of legs tight

keep elbows and shoulders in line

lean slightly forward

keep arms within peripheral vision

don't lock the elbows

don't fold arms too tightly

use internal resistance

annotations provide extra cues, tips and insights

>> from the top down

from the top down >>

9

The step-by-steps Work from left to right as you follow the step-by-step exercises. Be certain you understand the beginning and end positions before progressing.

the gatefold shows all the main steps of the programme

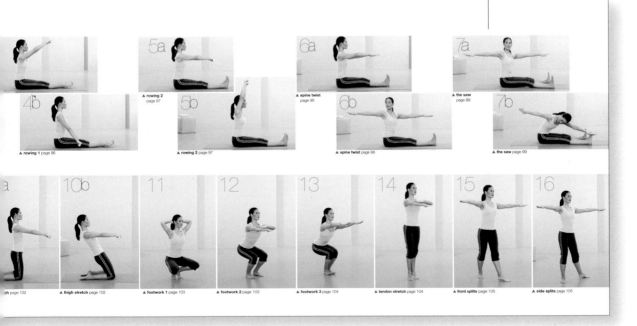

▲ rowing 1 page 96

5a ▲ rowing 2 page 97

▲ rowing 2 page 97

6a ▲ spine twist page 98

▲ spine twist page 98

7a ▲ the saw page 99

▲ the saw page 99

ch page 102

▲ thigh stretch page 102

▲ footwork 1 page 103

▲ footwork 2 page 103

▲ footwork 3 page 104

▲ tendon stretch page 104

▲ front splits page 105

▲ side splits page 105

>> **what you need** to start

People spend so much time getting ready to exercise that many never actually do it. I have a badge that reads, 'I'm in no shape to exercise'. This is an unfortunate and all-too common sentiment. Contrary to popular belief, it is unnecessary to prepare for exercise. You simply must decide to begin.

You will need nothing more than some 1kg (2lb) hand weights and a well-padded mat. Since some rolling exercises can cause bruising on an unpadded surface, many yoga mats may be unsuitable. Instead, choose a mat specifically for Pilates. Finally, keep a towel handy as well as some water, and you'll be ready to go.

Clothing is next. I once had a client with knock knees who happened to be wearing trousers with a seam down the front of the legs. Without thinking, I asked her to position her legs so that the seam was perfectly straight. Voilà! Her legs were better aligned and most importantly, she could see it herself. Whenever possible, select clothing with stripes or visible seams. You'll immediately notice asymmetries and will naturally correct them.

Pilates is normally performed barefoot. However, studios and health clubs often institute a footwear requirement. Bare feet are fine for the home, but for other settings, look for socks with grips to reduce slippage and protect your feet. There are even socks with compartments for each toe. Whatever you select, be sure to avoid slippery socks or cumbersome shoes that might reduce foot mobility.

Where to work out

The single largest impediment to any exercise programme is inconvenience, so find yourself a

A proper Pilates mat, a hand towel and some small hand weights (1kg/2lb) are all you need to begin these Pilates programmes. Be sure you have a clear space to work out.

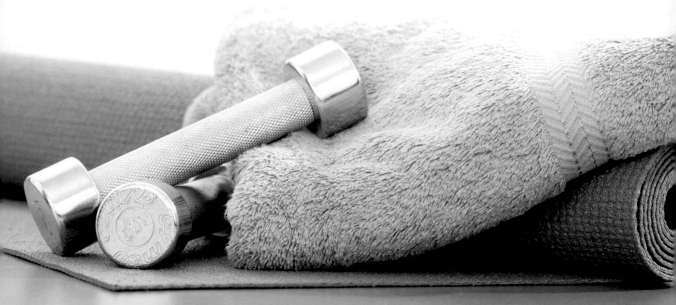

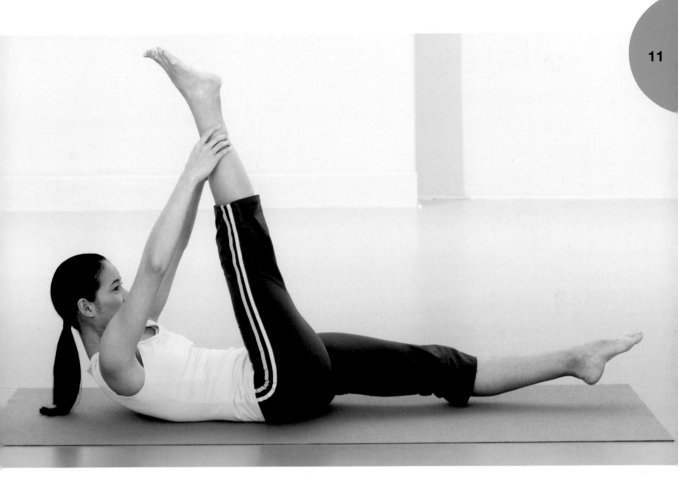

place that is easy to get to and a time that is convenient for your schedule. Pilates can be done anywhere you have enough room to stretch out on a mat. You can practise at a gym or at home. You can even practise on a lawn or beach, as long as you have an appropriate mat.

The safety instinct

Have you ever heard a little voice inside your head cautioning you to stop what you were doing? Did you listen? If you did, you are probably naturally intuitive about safety. For the rest of us, developing that intuition will be largely trial and error. To keep you working out safely, here are some guidelines:

1 Begin with just one programme.
2 Remember to hydrate. By the time you feel thirsty, you are already dehydrated.
3 Learn to distinguish between effort and pain. Effort is OK, pain is a signal to stop.
4 If something doesn't 'feel' right, stop.

Clothing can be a visual aid as you work out. Selecting attire with stripes can help you establish good alignment and make improvements to your form.

>> tips for getting started

- **Don't waste time** getting ready to exercise. You are ready. Just begin.

- **If a mat is not readily available** use some folded blankets or large towels instead. Plush carpeting can also be a suitable workout surface.

- **Find a time of day** when your energy is at its lowest. Just lying down for one exercise will get your blood flowing and will give you an energy burst.

>> **pilates** from the inside out

Therapists train their patients to become self-aware. This is a significant step towards mental and emotional wellbeing. Similarly, exercise instructors teach you to become physically self-aware. By recognizing your habits and body mechanics, you can embark upon a path of physical health and wellbeing.

Your body is amazing. The co-ordination of events required for simple actions such as bending your knee or opening your hand is astonishing, yet they happen without us noticing a thing.

By contrast, Pilates teaches your mind to train your body very consciously. During the programmes you will continually be required to recognize your positions, make adjustments and note how you feel. In addition, you must also be focused on the order of exercises, so that you can anticipate and prepare for the next move.

This 'mind–body' connection often suggests a workout that is neither physical nor rigorous, but Pilates is both. Just because we think our way through Pilates does not make it less taxing on the muscles. In fact, just the opposite is true. In the words of the late Frederick Schiller, 'It is the mind itself that builds the body.' Joseph Pilates (see pp122–123) was quite fond of this saying.

Learning new patterns

Our brains are built to learn new patterns. As we learn new skills, connections between previously unconnected brain cells are formed. Repetition is key. Each time you do a correct abdominal curl you are building a connection that makes it easier to do correctly the next time. In sum, 'cells that fire together, wire together'.

Pilates trains this mind-to-body dialogue. You will learn to direct your actions on a gross motor scale as well as a fine motor scale so your results will be amplified and expedited.

> ## >> **just make it** happen
>
> - **Pay attention to your body** throughout your day. Self-awareness is key to good health. If you watch how you move, your exercise routine will improve.
>
> - **Exercise is an activity.** It is not something that happens to you – you make it happen.
>
> - **It requires more energy to avoid** something than simply to do it. Don't waste any time making excuses. Just hit the mat and get started!

Your Pilates body

As you read this book and progress through the workouts, you will find instructions for and mentions of specific parts of your body. The chart opposite is a handy reference guide to them. For ease of use, we have chosen lay-person terms rather than anatomical ones. Names and labels allow your mind to grasp more effectively what is required of you, so become familiar with them and use them as you move through your workout. Think of the chart as a map for your mind.

Remember these simple names for your body parts. Learning about your anatomy will help you identify trouble spots as well as areas of strength in your body.

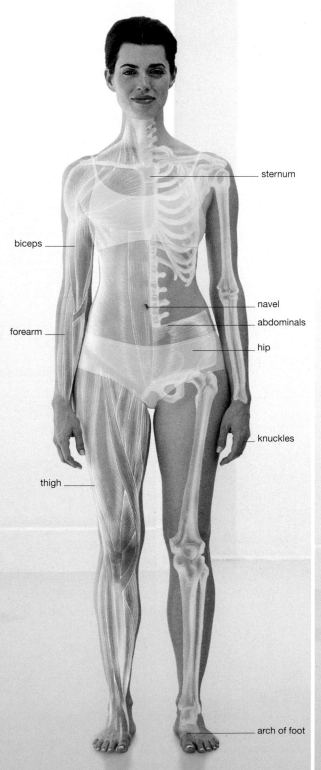

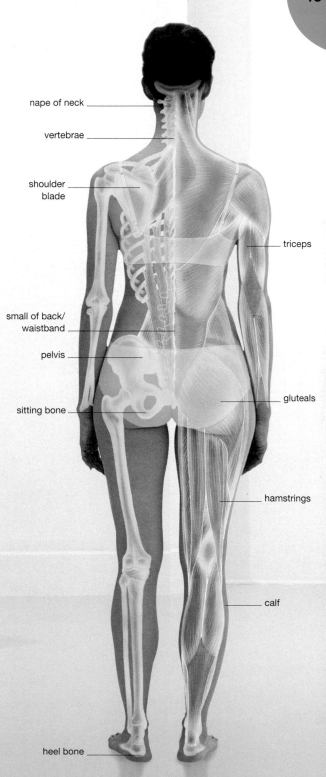

sternum

biceps

forearm

navel

abdominals

hip

knuckles

thigh

arch of foot

nape of neck

vertebrae

shoulder blade

triceps

small of back/ waistband

pelvis

gluteals

sitting bone

hamstrings

calf

heel bone

>> **pilates** concepts

Your Pilates technique and form can constantly be improved upon. Just as musicians must rehearse tirelessly, so Pilates will only get better as you train. Think of it as a language. First you learn the words, then some phrases, and finally you work on your accent. Let's begin here with your first Pilates words.

Before you can start on the mechanics of Pilates, there are six fundamental principles that you should become familiar with. These principles give substance and purpose to the workouts and help you learn to integrate your workout into your life so you begin to feel healthy and strong. Remember, the benefits of Pilates are meant to extend well beyond the actual workout.

Control

This is the primary principle of the system. In his time, Mr Pilates called his method 'Contrology'. His focus on controlled movement was a result of his years of blending Eastern and Western disciplines. As you work out, control your muscles, your positions and your tempos. Your body is your tool and by exerting control over it, it will produce better and better results.

Centring

This is a somewhat vague principle to many people. The idea is that all movement begins from your centre. I'm of the mind that Pilates was really drawing on the principle that you must 'stabilize before you mobilize'. In Pilates we brace or stabilize the core and then mobilize the limbs. Beyond that, there is an energetic component in working from your centre. It's as though you were able to harness and then project out through the limbs all of the energy and activity going on in your internal organs. Centring is akin to saying you should work from the inside out.

> ## >> **tips for** surefire success
>
> - **Don't over-analyse the work.** Pilates is complicated but it's meant to be a moving system. Keep moving at all costs.
>
> - **Working out is an extension of your life.** Put the same effort into it that you would into anything else.
>
> - **Don't work out – work in!** Inner work shapes the outer body.
>
> - **Never say die.** If an exercise is easy, you're not working hard enough.
>
> - **Don't ask what** an exercise is good for. Mr Pilates said, 'It's good for the body.'

Concentration

Concentration is key to Pilates. Without focused concentration, any exercise can only be moderately beneficial. Concentration elevates your intensity and so takes your results up to a far higher level.

Precision

This is the fourth principle and just as many of the other principles apply globally, so 'precision' serves as an umbrella for this whole list. Attention to the smallest detail is what makes Pilates so effective.

Breath

Breathing is a focus of the Pilates work. Many people come to Pilates because they have heard that it is a breathing technique. You will learn step-by-step breathing in these programmes but it is not their focus. As a general rule, inhale to prepare for a movement and exhale as you execute it.

Flow of movement

This is an element that comes later in the practice but can be incorporated early on. As you learn each exercise, be sure to perform it in a seamless, flowing manner. Eventually you'll work on creating one long routine.

Minimum of movement

Other ideas and concepts, such as symmetry, balance and integration arise as instructors make their own contributions to Pilates. All of these are applicable but Mr Pilates clearly intended his work to be succinct, so when establishing its main tenets, he chose only the key moves and critical concepts. This working list of six incorporates all the dozens of ideas and concepts at play in Pilates.

Off the floor and out the door

Now that you've learned the six principles, think about how they apply to real life. Concepts such as control, precision or breath can be applied to your life anywhere and anytime. Your workout should be a microcosm of how you live. If you never did any of these programmes, you could still embark upon a brand-new lifestyle simply by incorporating these key principles.

Working out on your own should be just as focused as working with a trainer. Learn to be your own teacher by cueing and correcting yourself constantly.

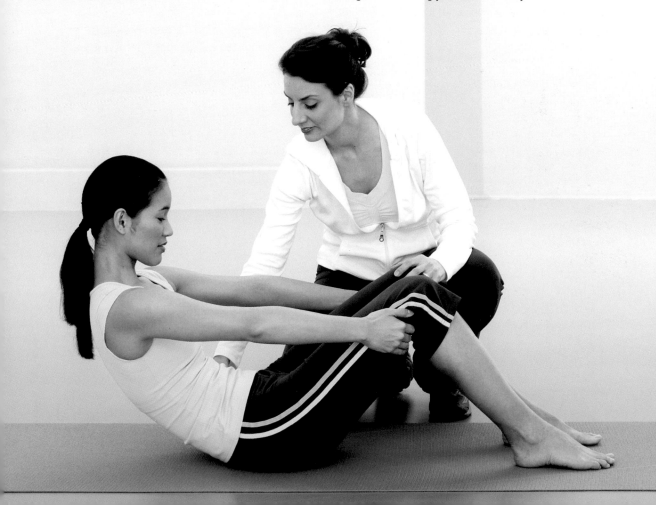

>> **pilates** top to tail

Now that we've covered the ideology of Pilates and the approach you will need to be successful, let's review the physical principles that are present throughout the programmes in this series. Certain elements of positioning are specific to Pilates. Let's start at the top of the body and work our way down.

To keep your neck well aligned during abdominal work, imagine resting your head on a raised support. The curve should be long and natural both front and back. Avoid any crunching or tightening around the throat.

Your breathing in Pilates needs to be specific. The abdominals must work in a contracted fashion at all times so your breathing must be redirected both upwards and outwards. Be aware that your lungs actually extend all the way above your collarbones. Practise breathing laterally, expanding the rib cage sideways as you inhale, and then contracting it inwards as you exhale.

Below the waist

Pilates teachers have several labels for the abdominals, including the core, the centre, and frequently, the powerhouse. No matter the tag,

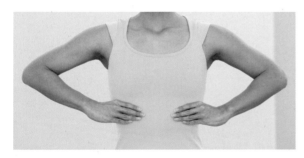

Practise breathing laterally with the hands on either side of the rib cage. On an inhale, the hands should pull apart.

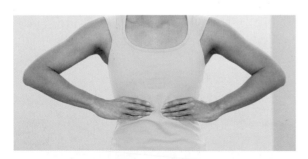

Exhale and feel the ribs narrowing. The hands draw together. Keep the abdominals tight.

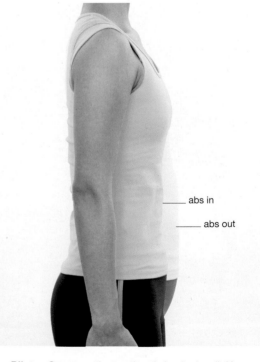

_____ abs in

_____ abs out

The Pilates Scoop activates the abdominal wall. Keep your waist lifted and narrowed. Never allow it to collapse.

your strength and control always spring from the centre of your torso. Your powerhouse specifically incorporates your abs, hips and buttocks as well.

The Pilates Scoop is the signature of the method. Even if you have difficulty pulling the abdominals inwards, you must never allow them to push outwards.

Optimal spinal alignment means positioning your spine to preserve its natural curves. To do this, when you are lying flat for abdominal exercises, try not to tuck or curl the lower back. Instead, aim to lengthen the spine. The end result should be strong, supportive abdominal muscles.

Additionally, when you are working your seat muscles or gluteals, think of 'wrapping' the muscles of the buttocks and thighs around towards the back. This will create a tightening and lifting of those muscles and will help to support your spine.

Pilates position or Pilates stance doesn't happen in the feet, although it looks as if it does. Working from your hips down, the gluteal muscles in your rear-end and in the backs of your thighs work together to rotate and wrap around. This causes a slight opening of the toes.

Perfect the details

As you work out, focus on your symmetry. Imagine your torso in a box from shoulders to hips. If your box is square, you are probably well aligned. You also need to work within your 'frame', which means keeping your limbs within your peripheral vision and never going beyond a comfortable joint range.

Never forget that Pilates is strength training. To maximize its benefits you must always work with resistance. Some resistance is provided by gravity and your positions. More important is the internal resistance you create. Your entire Pilates routine should incorporate this internal resistance.

Opposition is a final but vital ingredient of your Pilates practice. For every action there is an equal and opposite reaction. Pilates is the same. As one side reaches, another side contracts. If you lift up, you also anchor down. By using direct opposition you will find the stability and strength in your core to build a better body.

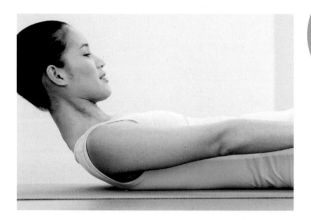

In abdominal work keep your neck lengthened and aligned. Don't force the chin down or tense the throat. Lifting the head comes from your abdominal strength.

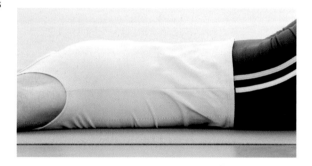

Performing exercises on your back can be tricky for your spine. When working your abdominals, keep your spine lengthened rather than curling it up underneath you.

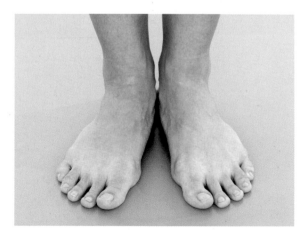

In Pilates stance the heels connect as the toes open. This is achieved by activating and rotating the buttock muscles and the muscles in the backs of the thighs.

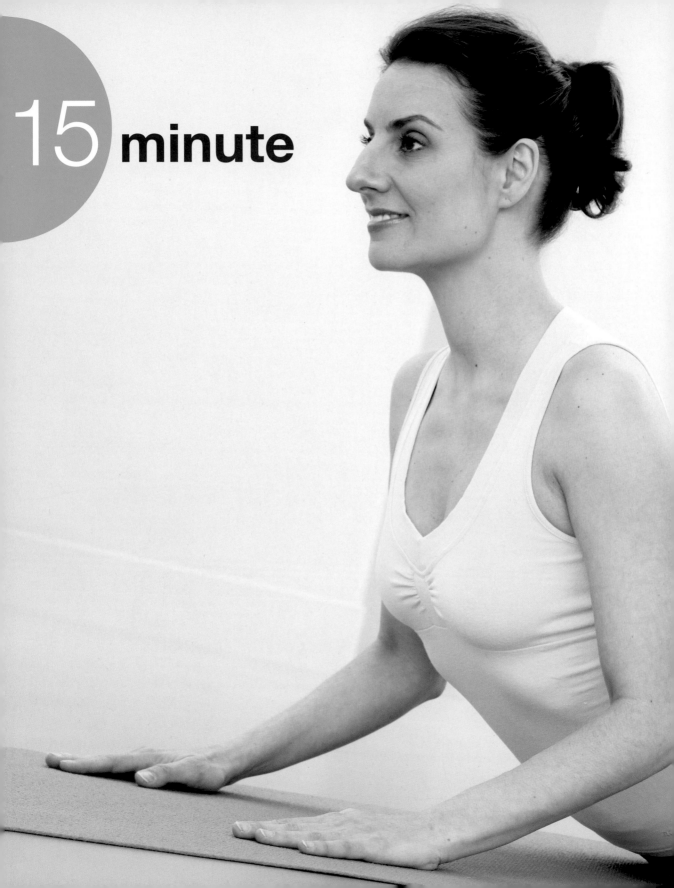

15 minute

Focus on control
Activate your powerhouse
Learn the classic routine

day by **day**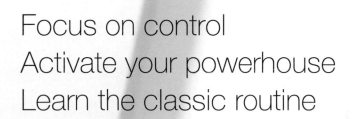

>> **day** by **day**

This programme is designed to be the first routine you learn. Perform it every day if possible. If you can only commit to one programme, this is your best choice. This classical sequence of movements contains all the benefits of the Pilates method and serves as a primer for all of your other programmes.

Your goal here is to learn how to move according to the six principles and the physical guidelines of Pilates (see pp14–17). We begin the programme with some specific abdominal recruitment exercises to get you breathing correctly and also to teach you to use your abdominals effectively. The remainder of the routine is as Mr Pilates developed it. We end with a rolling exercise which may be challenging at first but will, with practice, be possible.

Starting and finishing

Practise the initiation of each move in several ways. First, scan your body parts for their positions and for any necessary adjustments. Second, before moving anything, take a breath. Finally, brace or activate your centre to stabilize your core and free your limbs to do their work.

To end an exercise, linger at the final moment as though you were posing for a photograph, but rather than freezing your body in space, try to exaggerate the important points. Go for a deeper stretch, a longer leg, a more scooped-out midsection. Then you can rest.

Transitions

Weaving your way from one exercise to another with elegance and precision is the goal. The images on the right illustrate proper transitioning through movements. Transition from sitting to lying through a curling-down movement, and from lying to sitting through a curling-up movement. If this is too difficult, simply roll onto your side to get down or up between movements.

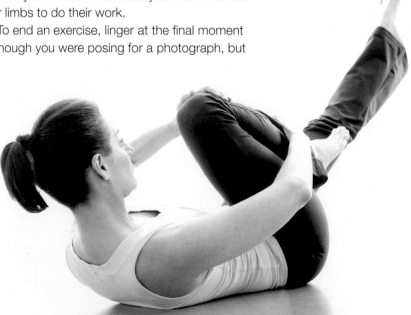

from **move** to move

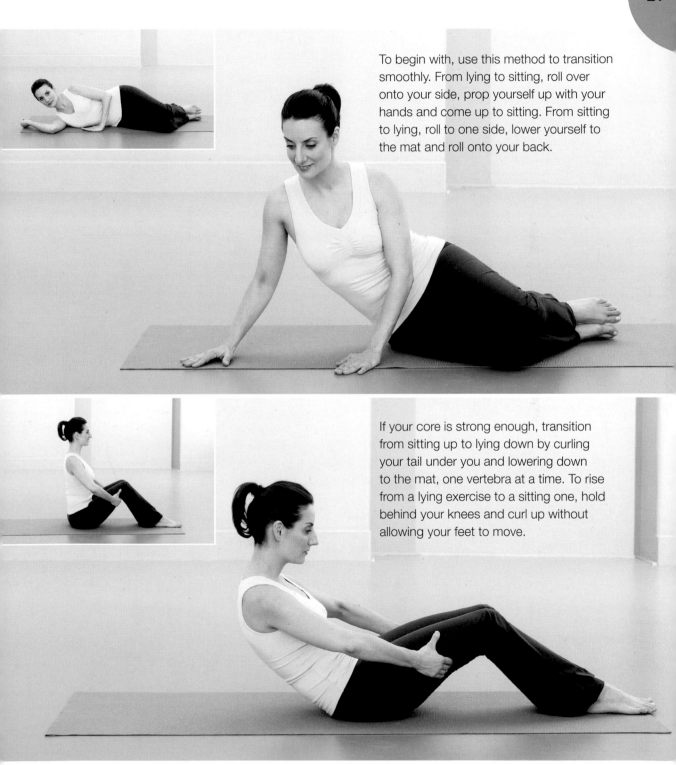

To begin with, use this method to transition smoothly. From lying to sitting, roll over onto your side, prop yourself up with your hands and come up to sitting. From sitting to lying, roll to one side, lower yourself to the mat and roll onto your back.

If your core is strong enough, transition from sitting up to lying down by curling your tail under you and lowering down to the mat, one vertebra at a time. To rise from a lying exercise to a sitting one, hold behind your knees and curl up without allowing your feet to move.

>> **abs wake-up**

1a Lie flat with your knees bent and your hands across your abdominals. Even lying flat, your posture should be perfect. Keep your neck long, your shoulders down and your 'box' square (see p17). Inhale deeply and let your abdominals expand. Your hands will lift as you do this.

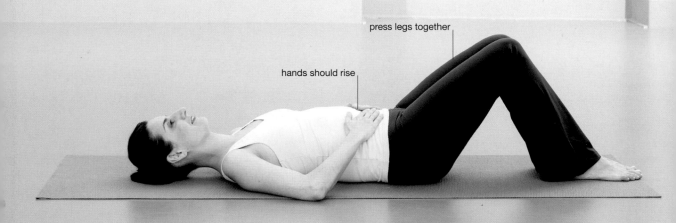

press legs together

hands should rise

1b Now exhale completely, emptying the lungs and sinking the abdominals. Don't crunch the midsection or hunch the shoulders. Just pull the belly in deeper, allowing the waist to hollow out. Repeat for 4 repetitions, exhaling longer and contracting deeper with each repetition.

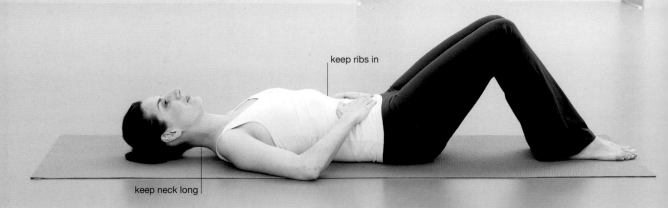

keep ribs in

keep neck long

>> abdominal curls

2a Extend your arms forwards so they hover just above the mat. Your feet remain firmly planted on the mat and your legs are pressed together. Your abdominals pull inwards and upwards. Prepare to curl up by inhaling.

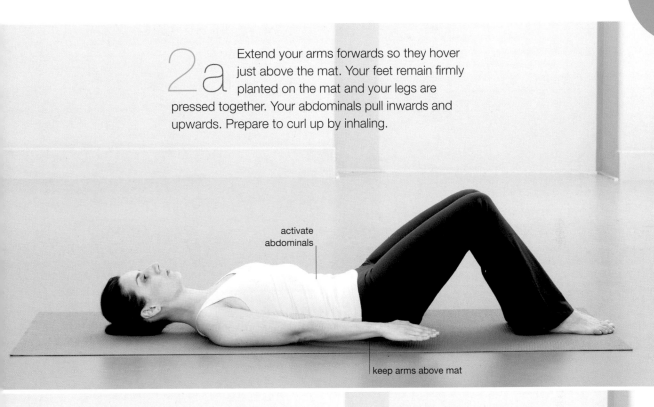

activate abdominals

keep arms above mat

2b Exhale, and without letting your abdominal wall expand, lift your head, neck and shoulders, curling up off the mat. Reach your arms longer and keep focused on your midsection. Lower down smoothly with an inhale. As you repeat, pull in your abdominals even further. Repeat 3 more times for a total of 4 repetitions.

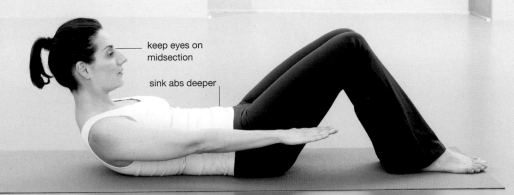

keep eyes on midsection

sink abs deeper

>> the hundred

3a Begin with both knees drawn into your chest. Curl your upper body up off the mat and reach your arms along your sides just above the mat. Pull in your abdominals.

pull abs in and up

keep hips flat on mat

3b Take both legs up to a 90° angle, with the shins parallel to the floor. Pump the arms up and down vigorously, breathing in for 5 pumps and out for 5 pumps. Continue until you reach 100, resting briefly if needed. Keep the abdominals deep and the torso still and strong.

point knees straight up

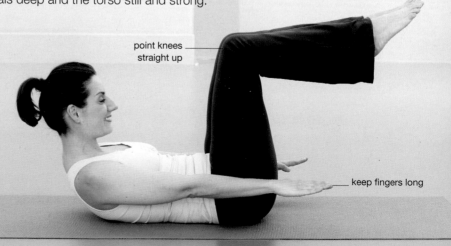

keep fingers long

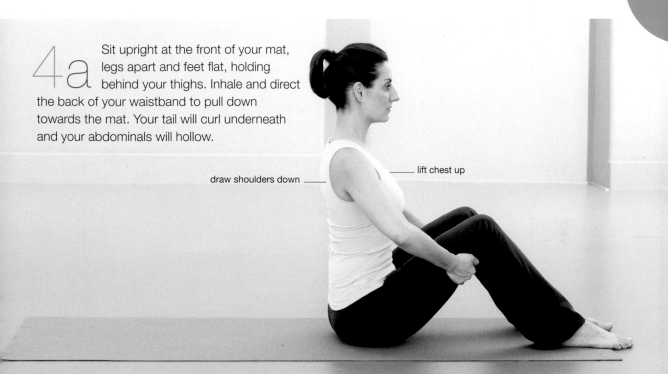

4a Sit upright at the front of your mat, legs apart and feet flat, holding behind your thighs. Inhale and direct the back of your waistband to pull down towards the mat. Your tail will curl underneath and your abdominals will hollow.

draw shoulders down _____ _____ lift chest up

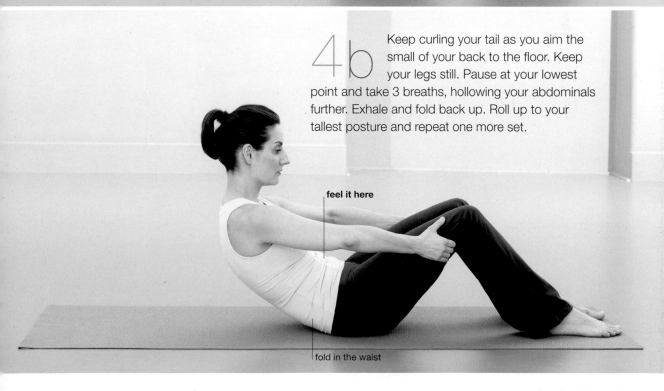

4b Keep curling your tail as you aim the small of your back to the floor. Keep your legs still. Pause at your lowest point and take 3 breaths, hollowing your abdominals further. Exhale and fold back up. Roll up to your tallest posture and repeat one more set.

feel it here

fold in the waist

>> single-leg circles

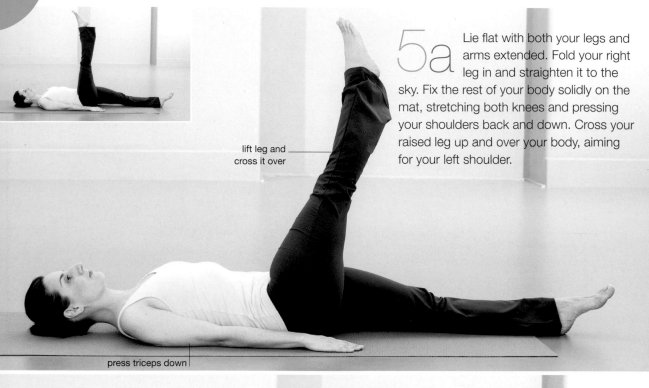

5a Lie flat with both your legs and arms extended. Fold your right leg in and straighten it to the sky. Fix the rest of your body solidly on the mat, stretching both knees and pressing your shoulders back and down. Cross your raised leg up and over your body, aiming for your left shoulder.

lift leg and
cross it over

press triceps down

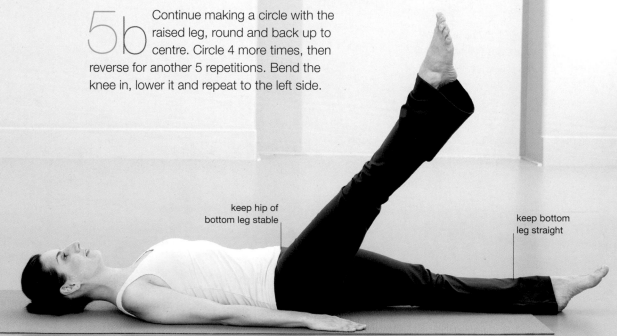

5b Continue making a circle with the raised leg, round and back up to centre. Circle 4 more times, then reverse for another 5 repetitions. Bend the knee in, lower it and repeat to the left side.

keep hip of
bottom leg stable

keep bottom
leg straight

6a Sit at the front edge of your mat, holding behind your thighs with your legs in the air. Keep your shins parallel to the floor. Hold your chest high and scoop your abdominals. Your elbows are open wide and your ankles are long.

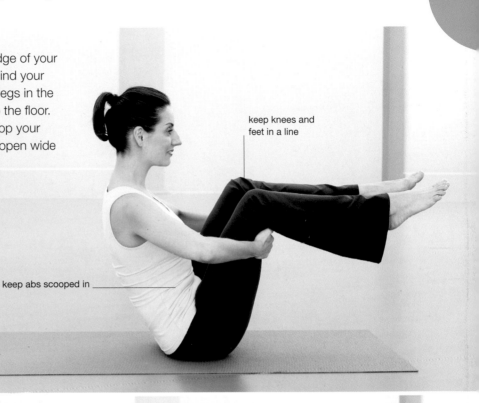

keep knees and feet in a line

keep abs scooped in

6b Tip your pelvis under you, then use your abs to ease back further. At your limit, pull your abs in further and fold your waist in, rounding forwards. Sit tall and repeat 3 more times. Lower your feet only after the last repetition.

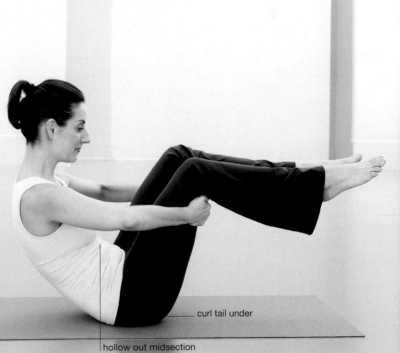

curl tail under

hollow out midsection

>> single-leg stretch

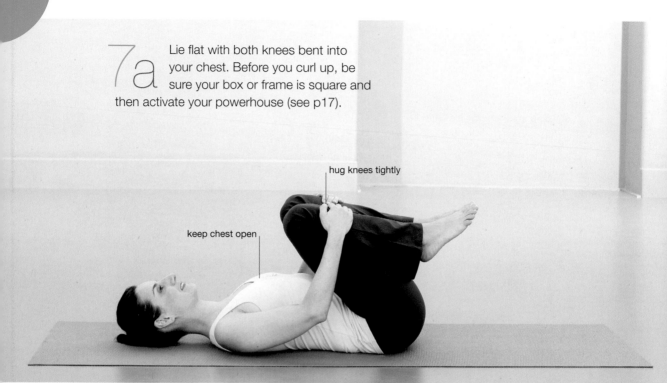

7a Lie flat with both knees bent into your chest. Before you curl up, be sure your box or frame is square and then activate your powerhouse (see p17).

hug knees tightly

keep chest open

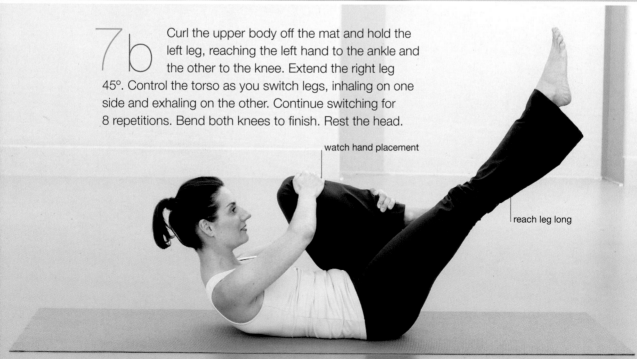

7b Curl the upper body off the mat and hold the left leg, reaching the left hand to the ankle and the other to the knee. Extend the right leg 45°. Control the torso as you switch legs, inhaling on one side and exhaling on the other. Continue switching for 8 repetitions. Bend both knees to finish. Rest the head.

watch hand placement

reach leg long

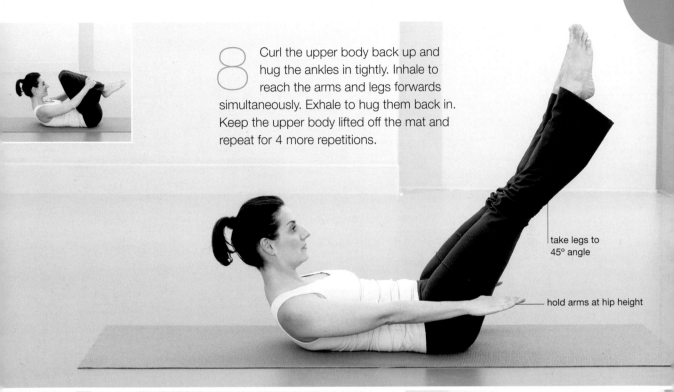

8 Curl the upper body back up and hug the ankles in tightly. Inhale to reach the arms and legs forwards simultaneously. Exhale to hug them back in. Keep the upper body lifted off the mat and repeat for 4 more repetitions.

take legs to 45° angle

hold arms at hip height

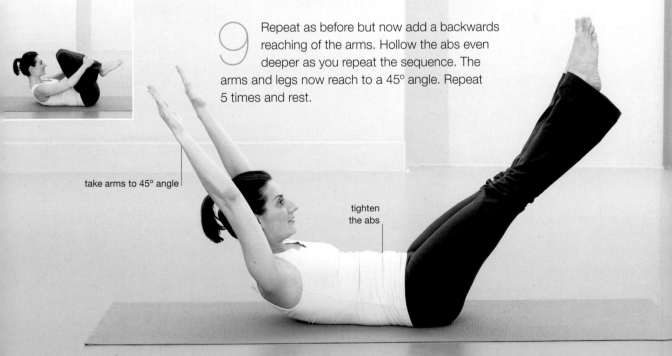

9 Repeat as before but now add a backwards reaching of the arms. Hollow the abs even deeper as you repeat the sequence. The arms and legs now reach to a 45° angle. Repeat 5 times and rest.

take arms to 45° angle

tighten the abs

>> spine stretch forward

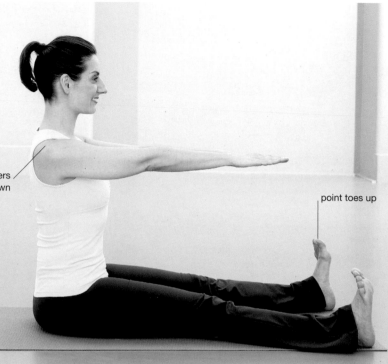

10a Sit tall at the front of your mat with your feet just wider than the mat. Extend both arms in front of you at shoulder height and flex your feet. Tighten your rear end and inhale so you feel as though you are rising up off the mat.

press shoulders down

point toes up

10b Exhale slowly and dive over, lowering your head and reaching forwards with your arms to stretch your back. As you round, pull back in your waist. Inhale to return to upright. Repeat 3 more times. After the final repetition, exaggerate your height, lengthening even taller.

dive head through arms

pull back in the waist

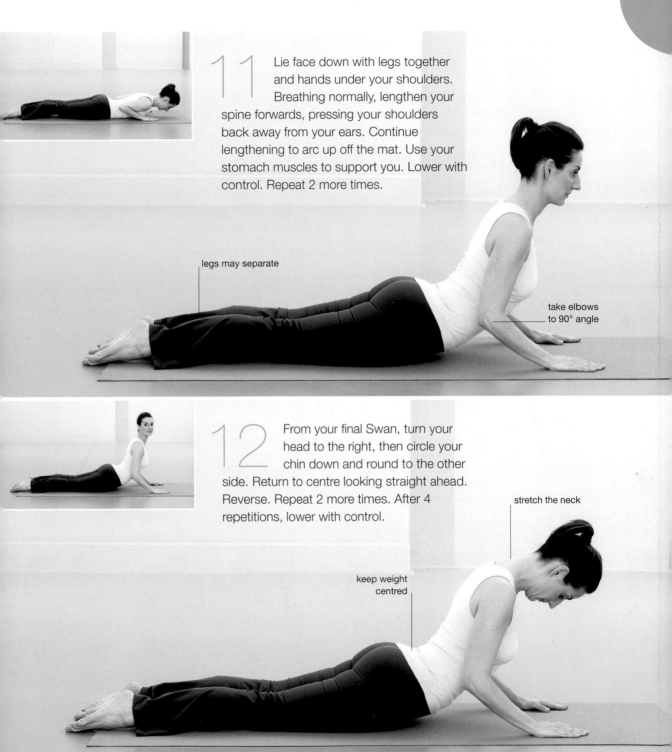

11 Lie face down with legs together and hands under your shoulders. Breathing normally, lengthen your spine forwards, pressing your shoulders back away from your ears. Continue lengthening to arc up off the mat. Use your stomach muscles to support you. Lower with control. Repeat 2 more times.

legs may separate

take elbows to 90° angle

12 From your final Swan, turn your head to the right, then circle your chin down and round to the other side. Return to centre looking straight ahead. Reverse. Repeat 2 more times. After 4 repetitions, lower with control.

stretch the neck

keep weight centred

>> child's pose/pelvic lift

13 Push back to sit on your heels with your back rounded, hands in front of you. Open your knees slightly to allow your upper body to sink deeper. Keep your abdominals lifted as you take 3 deep breaths. With each inhale, try to stretch and release your lower-back muscles. With each exhale, draw your navel even higher upwards. After 3 deep breaths, roll up to a kneeling position.

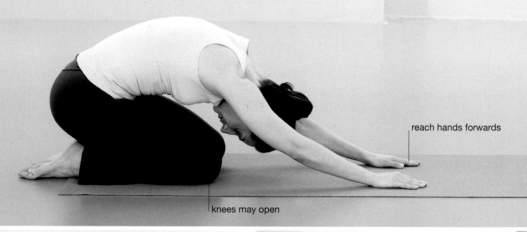

reach hands forwards

knees may open

14 Lie with knees bent and legs hip-width apart. Feel your chest open, shoulders back and spine long. Inhale and raise your hips without arching your back. Exhale and lower down, one vertebra at a time. Repeat 3 more times, increasing the articulation of your spine each time.

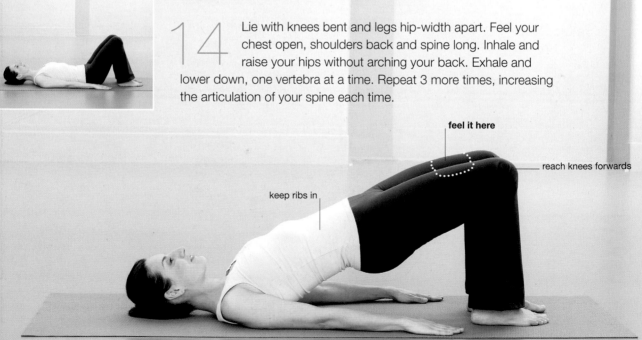

feel it here

reach knees forwards

keep ribs in

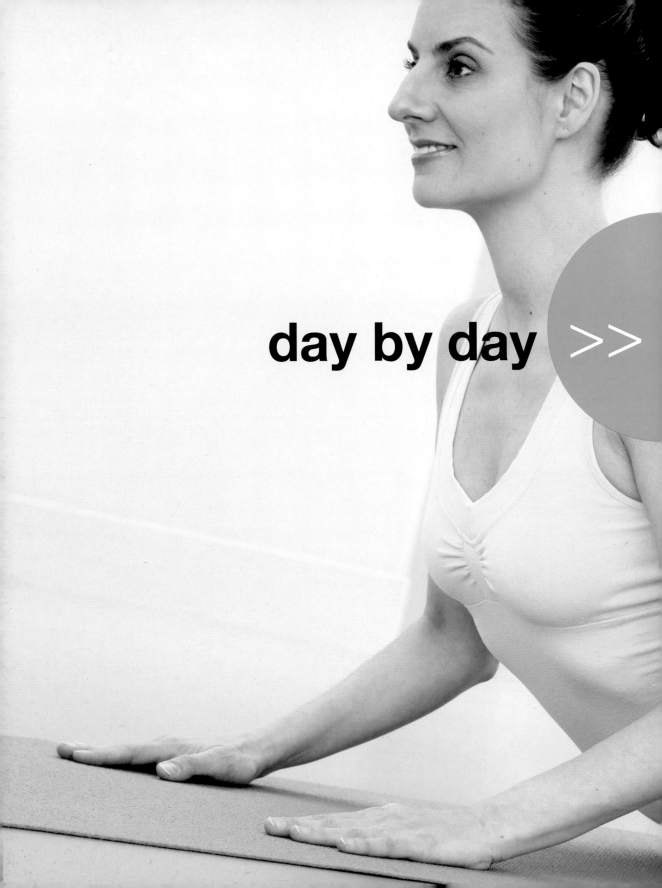

day by day >>

summary day by day

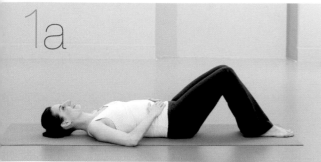

▲ **Abs Wake-up** page 22

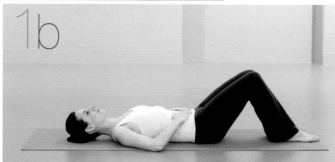

▲ **Abs Wake-up** page 22

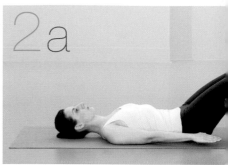

▲ **Abdominal Curls** page 23

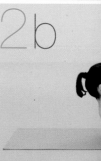

▲ **Abdominal Curls**

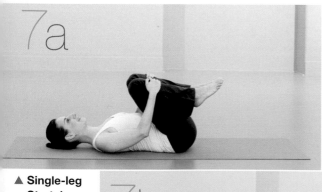

▲ **Single-leg Stretch** page 28

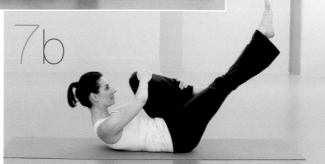

▲ **Single-leg Stretch** page 28

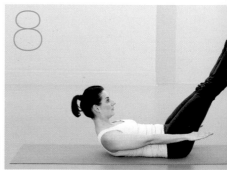

▲ **Double-leg Stretch 1** page 29

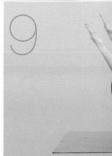

▲ **Double-leg Stretc**

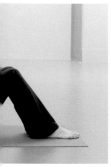

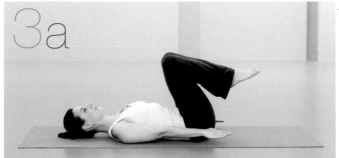

3a

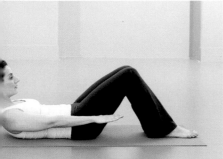

▲ **The Hundred** page 24

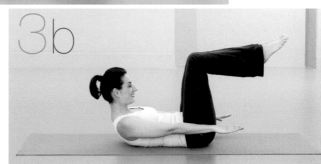

3b

page 23

▲ **The Hundred** page 24

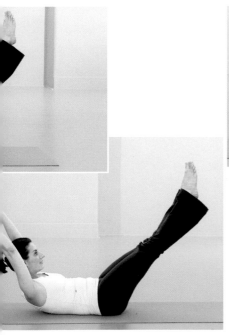

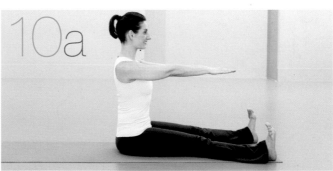

10a

▲ **Spine Stretch Forward** page 30

10b

h 2 page 29

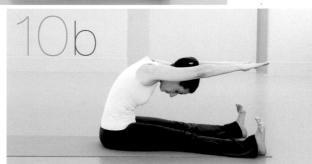

Spine Stretch Forward page 30

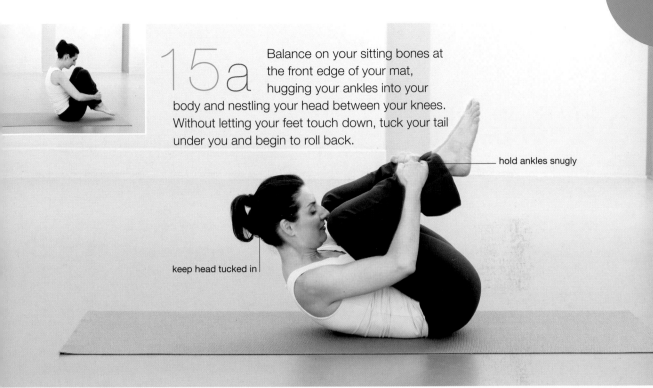

15a

Balance on your sitting bones at the front edge of your mat, hugging your ankles into your body and nestling your head between your knees. Without letting your feet touch down, tuck your tail under you and begin to roll back.

hold ankles snugly

keep head tucked in

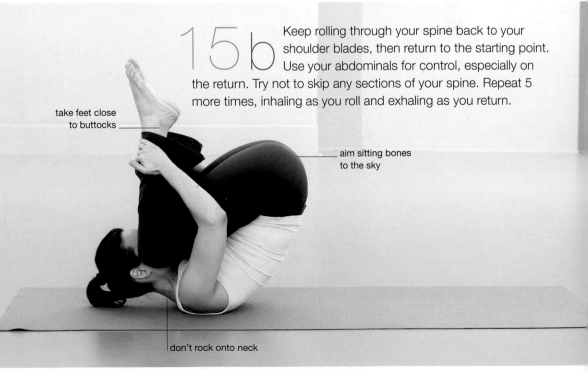

15b

Keep rolling through your spine back to your shoulder blades, then return to the starting point. Use your abdominals for control, especially on the return. Try not to skip any sections of your spine. Repeat 5 more times, inhaling as you roll and exhaling as you return.

take feet close to buttocks

aim sitting bones to the sky

don't rock onto neck

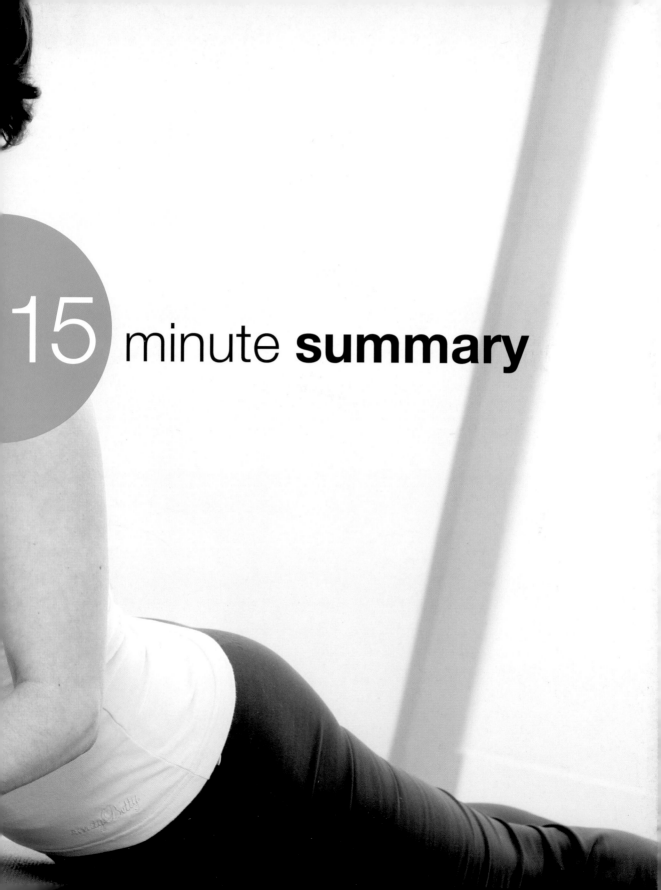

15 minute **summary**

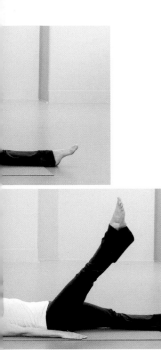

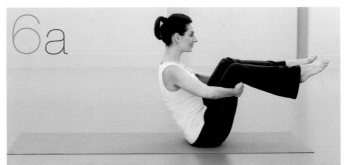

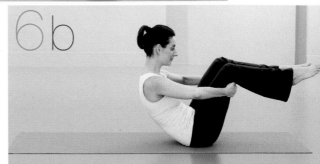

▲ **Rolling Preparation** page 27

▲ **Rolling Preparation** page 27

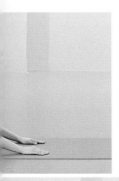

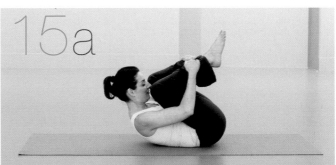

▲ **Rolling Like a Ball** page 33

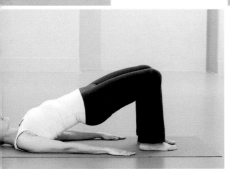

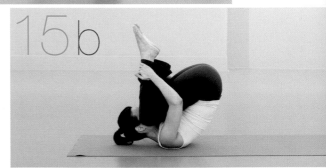

▲ **Rolling Like a Ball** page 33

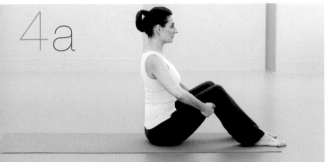

▲ **The Roll-down**
page 25

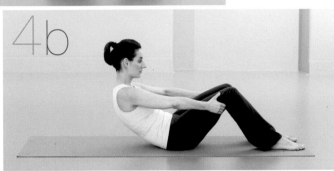

▲ **The Roll-down** page 25

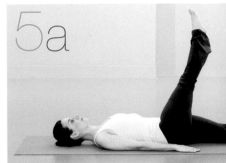

▲ **Single-leg
Circles**
page 26

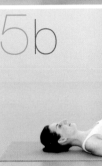

▲ **Single-leg Circle**

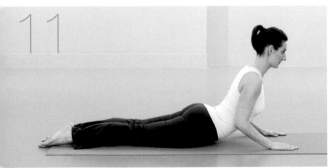

▲ **The Swan**
page 31

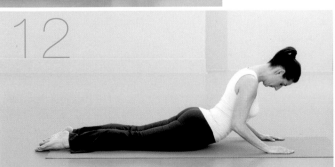

▲ **Neck Roll** page 31

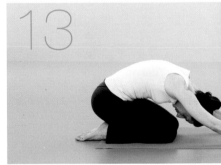

▲ **Child's Pose**
page 32

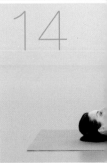

▲ **Pelvic Lift** page 3

>> **day by day** extras

The most important thing about this programme is making sure you do it.

Once you have the routine memorized, it will take less time and effort to

perform. To help you commit the order to memory, try writing the names

of the exercises down or singing them along to a familiar tune.

>>   Checklist

Be sure to scan your moves for evidence of the six principles at work. The choreography of each move is less important than the quality of those movements.

• Did you transition smoothly between exercises using minimal movement while you were performing this programme?

• Have you accomplished the 'scoop' of the abdominals to draw the muscles inwards instead of distending them?

• When curling up, were you able to contract the abdominals fully without allowing any pushing outwards?

• During the Hundred did you manage to keep your upper body fixed at one height, resisting any shaking in the body?

• For the Single-Leg Circles, the hips must remain stable. Were you able to accomplish this?

• Were you able to isolate the pelvis in the Rolling Preparation so that no other body parts were moving?

• The Spine Stretch Forward should be performed as though your body were fixed against a wall and the upper back were peeling away from it. Did you feel that?

• The Pelvic Lift is a variation of a Pilates equipment exercise known as the Breathing. Were you able to articulate your spine fully as you lowered your hips back to the mat?

• Rolling like a Ball is an exercise in control. Are you able to sustain your balance for a moment between each repetition?

>> Modify/Adjust

It will benefit you more to perfect your form in a less advanced move than to force your body past its comfort zone. Modify as necessary.

• Change the bottom leg to a bent-knee position during the Single-Leg Circles.

• Alter your position to separate the legs slightly when lying on your stomach to alleviate lower-back pressure.

• Lower the head to avoid neck strain during exercises where the head is raised.

• Hold behind your knees rather than around the ankles.

>> Challenge

As you incorporate challenges, do so incrementally. This workout is meant to stay with you for a lifetime.

• Remember to linger at the end of each exercise to perfect your position even more for optimal results.

• Try to increase the resistance by creating internal pressure in your muscles as they push and pull against gravity.

• Vary the tempo to go slower during the hardest parts of each exercise – don't throw it away.

• Work to extend the legs a bit lower yet still remain scooped during the Single and Double-Leg Stretch.

• Use the curling-up transition rather than rolling through one side.

>> Trainer tips

The goal of this programme is to get you acquainted with your body. Focus your attention on problem areas within exercises.

• Connectivity is key. Stop moving between exercises and your body forgets that it is working out. No matter what – keep moving.

• Every movement has a counter-movement, so if you twist your torso you'll find one side is pulling backwards while the other pulls forwards. Pay attention to these naturally opposing moments in each exercise.

• When curling up, imagine four points at your ribs and hips and draw them together, sinking your abdominals.

15 minute

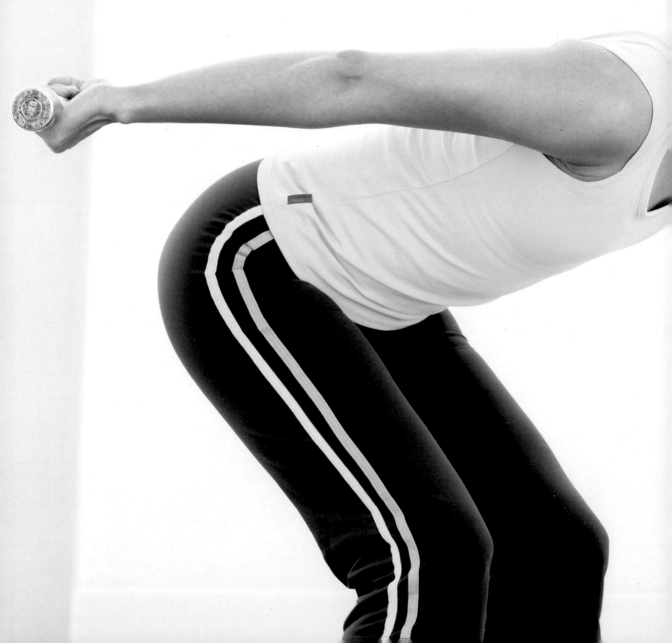

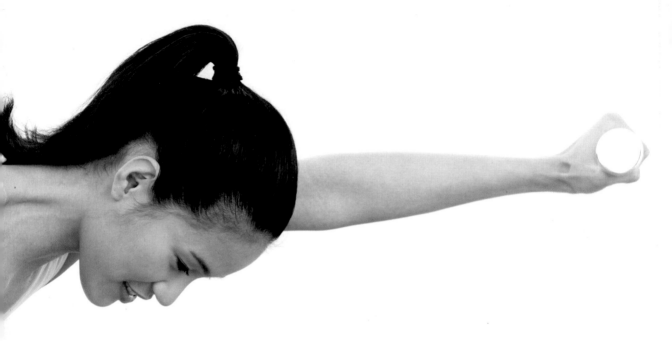

from the
top down >>

Focus on centring
Activate your Pilates box
Learn Pilates with weights

>> **from the** top down

This programme is comprised of standing exercises and is performed almost entirely with hand weights. I've structured the routine to show that Pilates is not confined to the mat. The programme you are about to do not only gets you upright, but also trains you to carry this work with you wherever you go.

We begin by standing for a series of arm and upper-body exercises, performed in Pilates stance. Then you move on to a flat-back series, which challenges your core, co-ordination and alignment, before coming upright again. Now the fun begins. The next set of exercises requires you to be utterly stable in movements that are targeted to bend you, shift you and shake you. You'll close the routine with some modified Pilates Push-ups and a historical breathing exercise – the Windmill.

Starting and finishing

To start off, you will need to establish a solid standing Pilates stance (see p17). The hamstrings will wrap tightly around the back and the buttocks will tense. For standing exercises in Pilates, there is a bit of an incline in the body. It's often described as 'leaning into the wind'. The position requires you to shift your weight slightly forwards towards the fronts, or balls, of the feet. You will sustain this position for each upright move in the programme.

At the end of this programme, we take a breathing reminder from a vintage exercise. Mr Pilates developed a hand-held device for improving breath control during the exercise. Today, we do it without but must remember to challenge our lungs to empty every drop of air before inhaling again.

Transitions

Linking the hand-weight exercises requires keeping your torso strong and stable and the arms moving fluidly. In the flat-back series, move from your flat

> ## >> **secrets** of success
>
> - **Use the Side Bends exercise** to emphasize opposition. As you reach up and away, anchor the opposite side of the body down into the ground.
>
> - **Push-ups are a great move** for working on spinal alignment. Once in your 'plank' position, arrange your spine in one solid line from your hips to the top of your head.
>
> - **Baby Circles** reinforce the idea of stability before mobility. The temptation to waver and vacillate as you circle must be resisted at all costs.

back into a rounded spine as though you were melting over your legs. From your lowest stretch, roll back up through your spine. In this series you will be shifting your body weight from upright, to bent over to rounded over. Whichever your body position, keep your weight centred through the middle of your feet. Don't sink back in the heels or rise up on the toes. Like all Pilates movements, these transitions are mindful and precise.

From the Top Down seems to focus on the upper body only. With practice, though, it becomes clear that every Pilates exercise is a full-body experience.

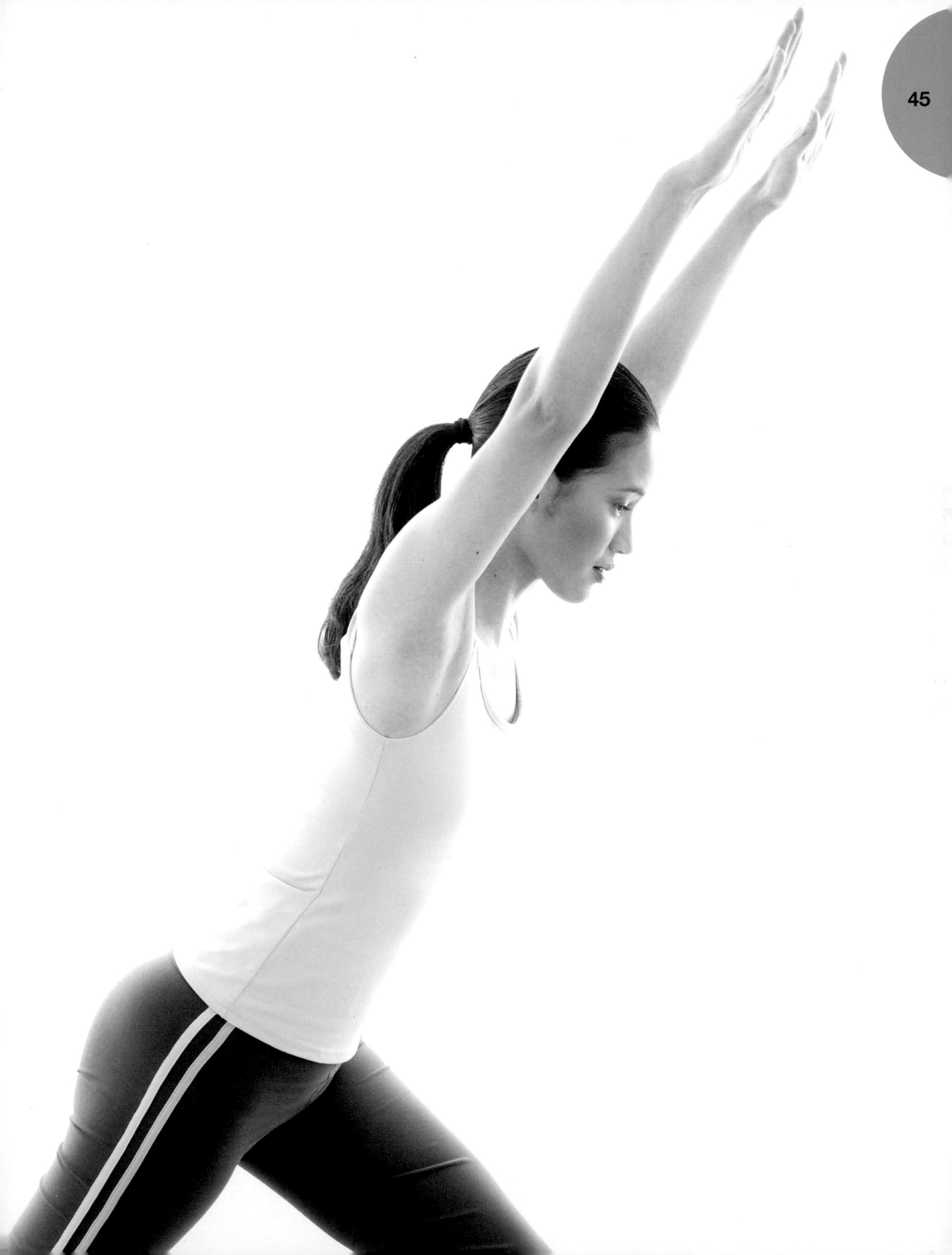

>> front curls

1a Holding a small weight in each hand, stand in Pilates position (see p17) with heels together and toes apart. Tighten the seat and draw the waistline inwards and upwards. Raise the arms forwards directly in front of you, in line with the shoulders, palms facing upwards. Keep the elbows long but not locked.

1b With internal resistance (see p17), bend the arms in past 90°. Be sure the elbows remain high as you bend them. Now open the arms out with the same resistance. Repeat 5 more times, inhaling to extend and exhaling to bend. On your last repetition, lower the arms smoothly down to your sides. Perform 6 repetitions.

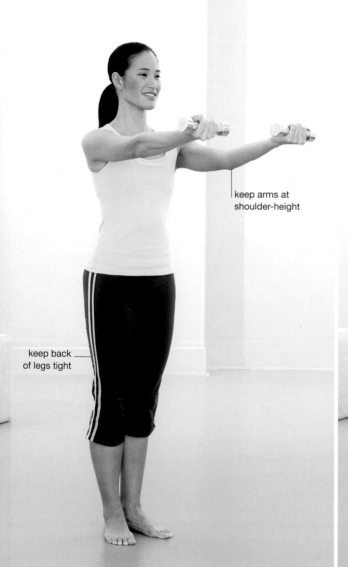

keep arms at shoulder-height

keep back of legs tight

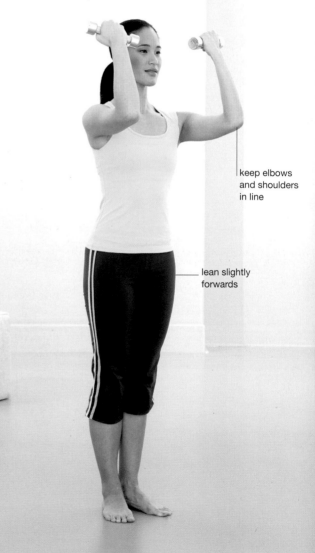

keep elbows and shoulders in line

lean slightly forwards

2a
Now raise both arms up sideways, just in front of the shoulders. Be sure to maintain a long spine and a strong core. Don't allow your posture to sink or collapse. Tighten the muscles of the buttocks so the lower half of you continues to work.

2b
Use resistance to bend the arms in past 90°. Use even more resistance to open the arms out. Be sure the elbows remain high as you bend and straighten. Repeat 5 more times, inhaling to extend and exhaling to bend. On your last repetition, lower the arms smoothly to your sides.

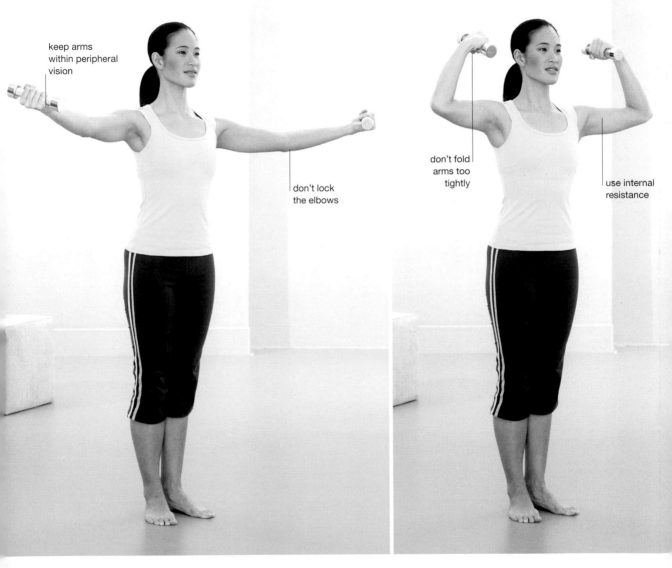

keep arms within peripheral vision

don't lock the elbows

don't fold arms too tightly

use internal resistance

>> **zip-ups**

3a Still holding the small weights, rotate the backs of the hands towards each other so the knuckles face each other. Scoop the abdominals up, tighten the backs of the legs and shift the weight a tiny bit forwards towards the fronts of the feet. Keep the heels flat as you do this. Inhale to prepare.

3b Exhale, open your elbows wide and pull the weights up under your chin, keeping your neck long and your shoulders relaxed. Lower the weights back down as though you were pushing something heavy away from you. Repeat 5 more times, inhaling to lift and exhaling to lower.

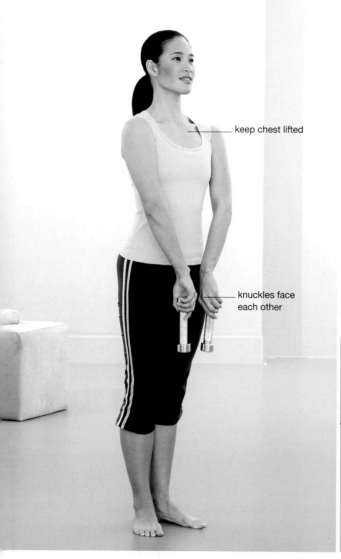

keep chest lifted

knuckles face each other

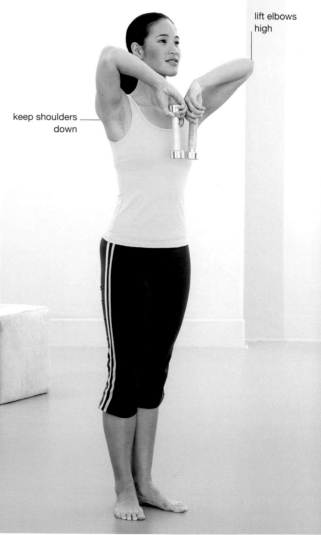

lift elbows high

keep shoulders down

4a Still holding the weights, place both of them behind your head at the nape of your neck. Tip your chin down slightly and be sure to keep your elbows open wide. Your feet remain in Pilates position with your legs pressed together tightly. Incline your body forwards as though you were 'leaning into the wind'.

4b Without locking the elbows, extend the arms overhead. Hold the powerhouse strong (see p17) and keep the fingers of each hand in contact with each other. Lower with resistance. Repeat 5 more times, exhaling to extend and inhaling to lower.

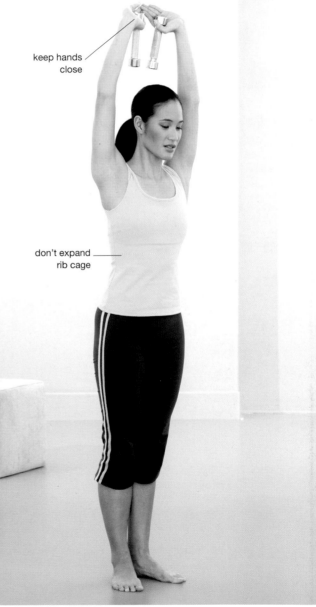

keep hands close

don't expand rib cage

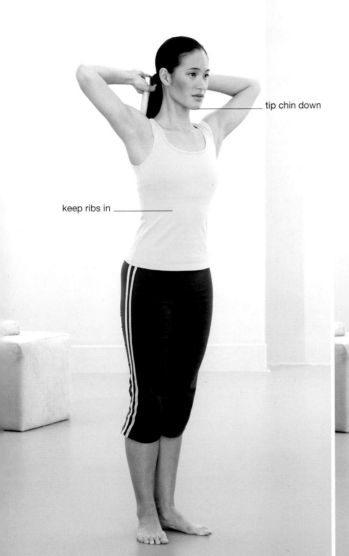

tip chin down

keep ribs in

>> **the boxing**

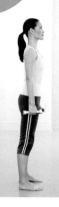

5a Open the feet into parallel, hip-width apart, and stand tall holding the weights. Bend both knees deeply and fold over the legs with a long flat back. Tuck the arms in by your sides, keeping the elbows tight to the body. Lift the abdominals without disrupting your posture. Inhale to prepare.

5b Exhale and simultaneously extend the right arm forwards and the left arm back in a boxing-like movement. Inhale to fold the arms back in. Continue, creating resistance and alternating sides for 3 full sets. Complete a total of 6 repetitions. To finish, round over the legs, stretching the back and legs. Slowly roll back up to standing.

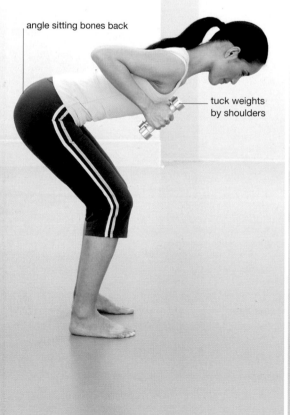

angle sitting bones back

tuck weights by shoulders

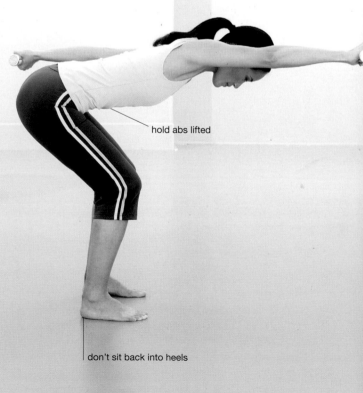

hold abs lifted

don't sit back into heels

>> the bug

6a Start by standing tall, holding the weights and with legs parallel. Bend your knees and fold over, keeping your spine long and flat. Frame your arms in a circle directly underneath you, bringing your fists towards each other. Lift your powerhouse and inhale to prepare.

6b Exhale and lift both arms to the sides of the room. Don't allow your body position to change as you do this. Inhale and lower your arms as though you were squeezing something together. Perform 2 more repetitions, then reverse your breathing and exhale to prepare for an additional 3 repetitions. Finally, round over your legs to release the spine.

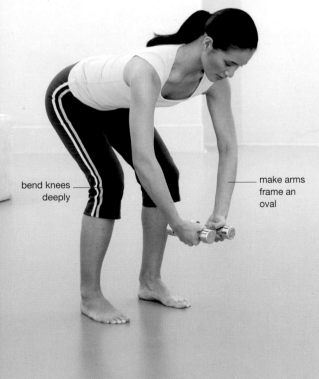

bend knees deeply

make arms frame an oval

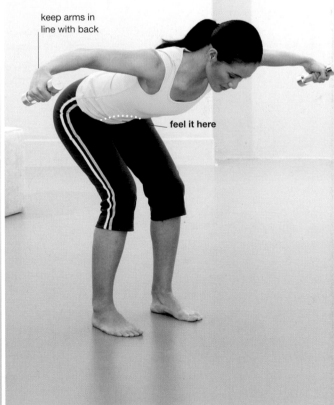

keep arms in line with back

feel it here

>> **triceps**

7a Holding the weights, stand tall with your legs parallel. Fold at your waist over your legs and tuck your arms in by your sides. Bring your elbows up a little higher than your back. Activate your abdominals and inhale to begin.

7b Exhale and extend both arms behind you, holding strong in your centre. Fold them back in slowly and with control, as though you were pulling something towards you. Repeat 5 more times. Stretch over your legs again before rolling up through your spine, one vertebra at a time.

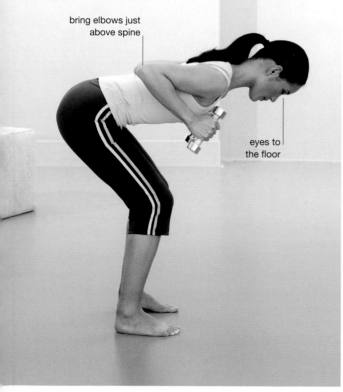

bring elbows just
above spine

eyes to
the floor

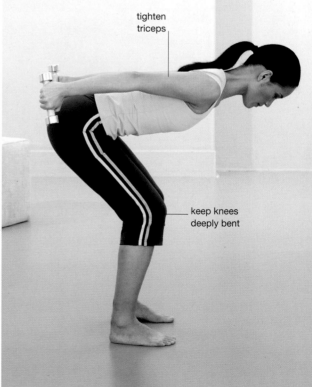

tighten
triceps

keep knees
deeply bent

>> **baby circles**

8a Standing in Pilates stance (see p17), hold your weights just in front of your legs on a slight angle. Shift your weight towards the fronts of your feet, leaning slightly forwards and tightening your gluteal muscles. Begin circling the arms 8 times, raising your arms higher with each circle until you are reaching overhead.

8b Reverse your circles, lowering down for 8 circles. Repeat another full set. Try not to shake or bounce your body as you circle your arms. Hold your torso strong and breathe naturally.

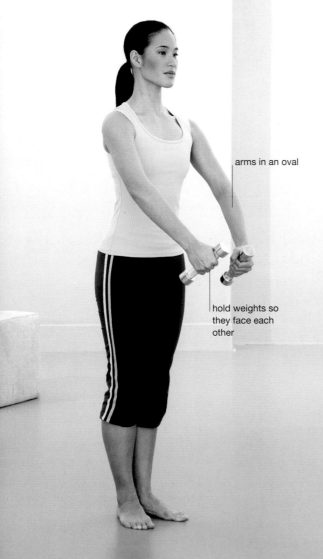

arms in an oval

hold weights so they face each other

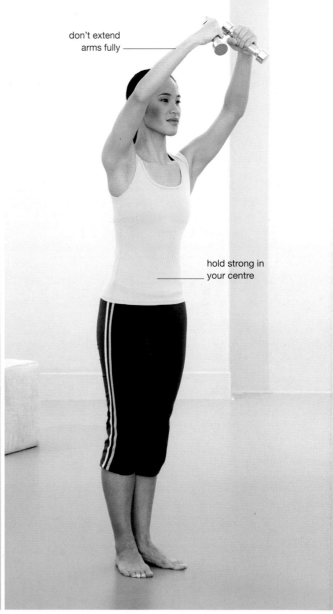

don't extend arms fully

hold strong in your centre

>> lunges

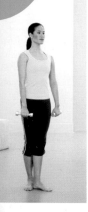

9a Holding the weights, stand with your feet in a 'Y', nestling the heel of your left foot into the arch of the right. Angle your body towards your left foot, holding the weights just in front of your thighs. Tighten the backs of your legs and draw your waist in and up. In a fencing-like motion, shoot your left leg out into a deep lunge position as your arms rise quickly up.

9b Shift back onto your straight leg, dragging your left foot back to your right foot as you lower your arms. Repeat 3 more times and switch sides.

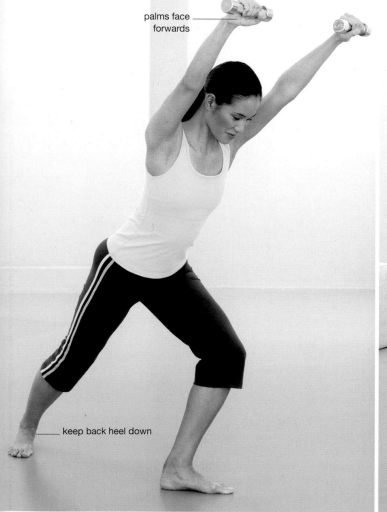

palms face forwards

keep back heel down

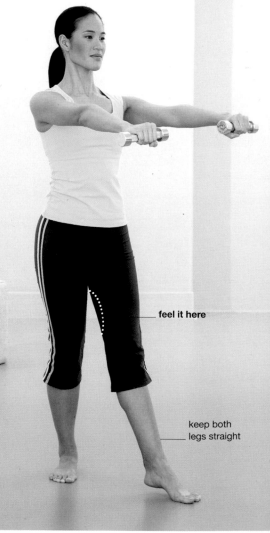

feel it here

keep both legs straight

>> side bend

10a Stand in Pilates stance and extend the right arm up towards the ceiling, hugging the arm against the side of the head. Inhale and lift even higher, arcing up and over to the left.

10b Bend up and away, reaching further over and allowing the bottom arm to hang loosely. Now return to the centre-line, resisting on the way up. Lower the arm down by your side and repeat to the left side. Perform 2 more sets for a total of 6 repetitions.

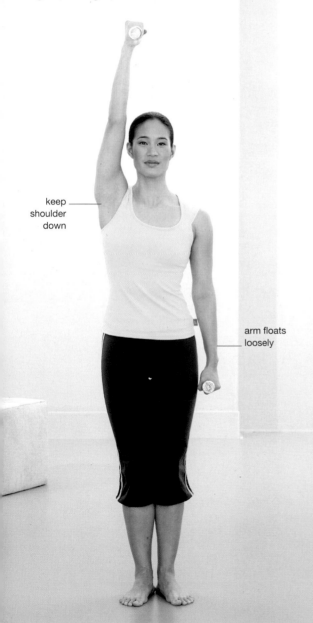

keep shoulder down

arm floats loosely

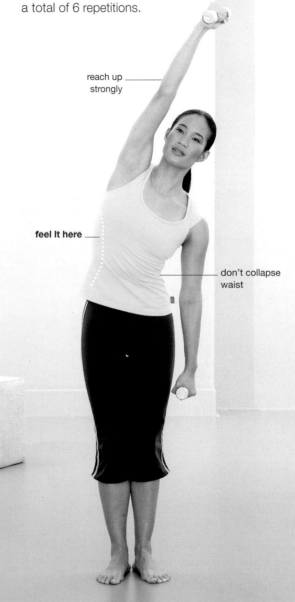

reach up strongly

feel It here

don't collapse waist

>> **push-ups**

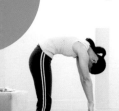

11a Stand upright in Pilates stance, tightening the backs of your legs. Reach your arms overhead for a breath, then dive over your legs, reaching for the floor and keeping your abdominals lifting. Walk your hands out until you are in a plank position and bend your knees up.

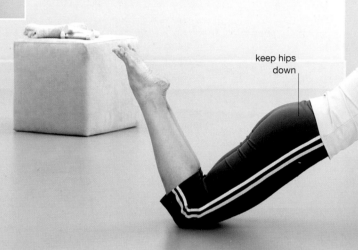

keep hips down

keep hands under shoulders

11b Open your elbows and lower your upper body up and down for 3 push-ups. Straighten your legs behind you, tuck your toes under and lift your hips, pressing back into your heels for a stretch. Carefully walk your hands back to your legs, stretch a moment and roll back up to standing. Repeat 1 more set for a total of 6 push-ups.

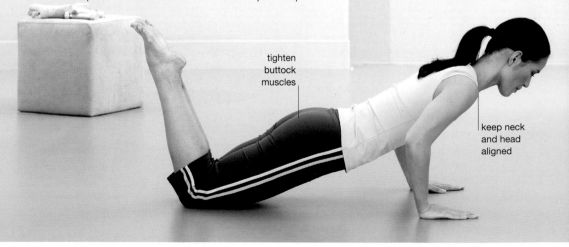

tighten buttock muscles

keep neck and head aligned

from the top down >>

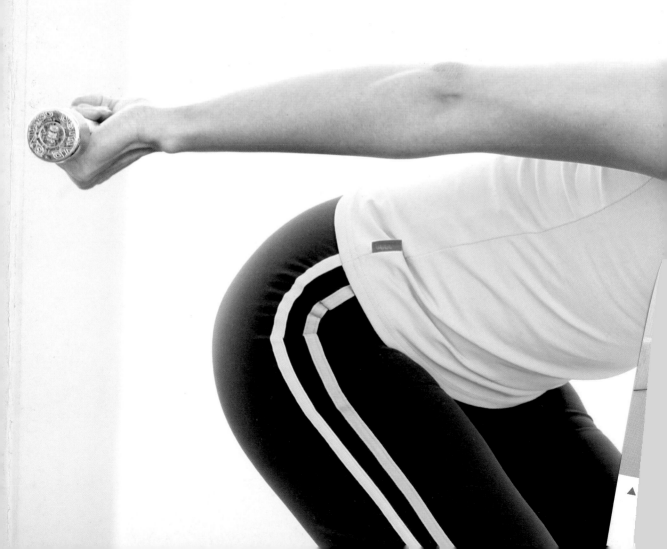

summary from the top down

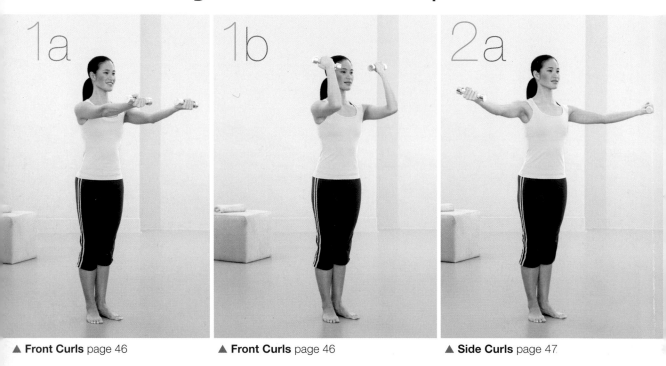

1a ▲ **Front Curls** page 46

1b ▲ **Front Curls** page 46

2a ▲ **Side Curls** page 47

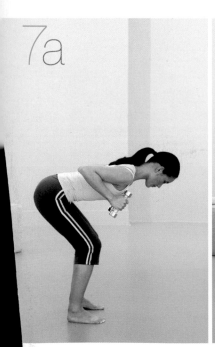

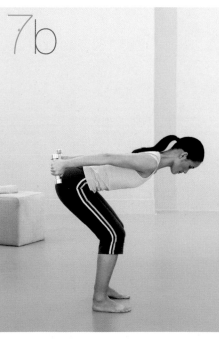

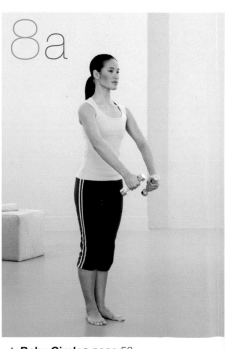

7a ▲ **Triceps** page 52

7b ▲ **Triceps** page 52

8a ▲ **Baby Circles** page 53

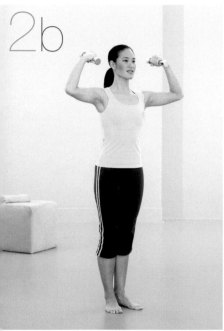

▲ **Side Curls** page 47

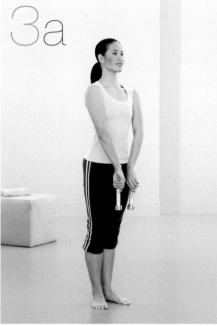

▲ **Zip-ups** page 48

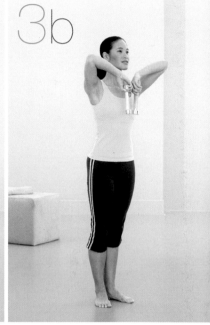

▲ **Zip-ups** page 48

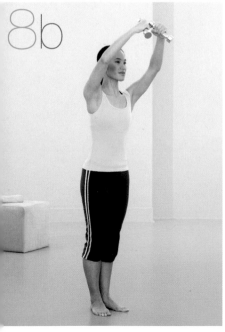

▲ **Baby Circles** page 53

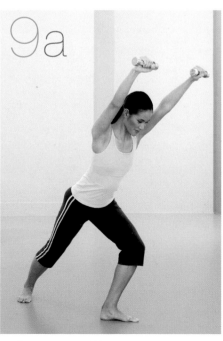

▲ **Lunges** page 54

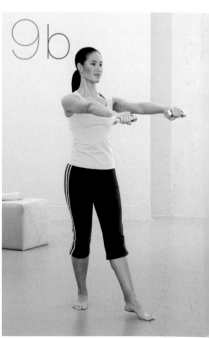

▲ **Lunges** page 54

12a Stand tall and envisage your spine as a wheel as you inhale. Exhale, tucking your head down and folding over your legs. Try to keep your weight shifted slightly forwards. Continue exhaling and rounding your spine down in a curling motion.

12b When you are folded over and have no air left, slowly inhale and uncurl the spine, rolling back up to standing. Repeat 2 more times, exhaling progressively longer each time. Finally, roll the shoulders back, lengthen the neck and stand tall.

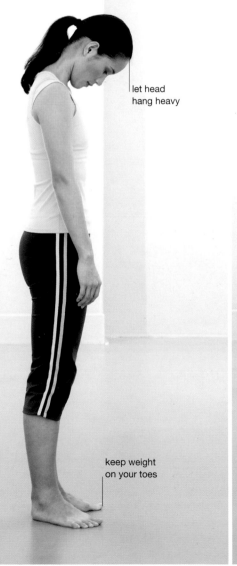

let head hang heavy

keep weight on your toes

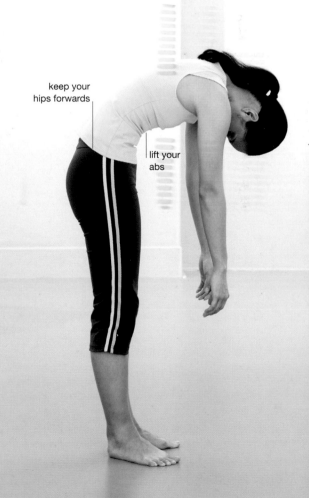

keep your hips forwards

lift your abs

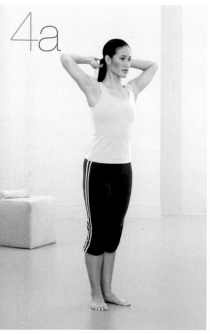

▲ **Salutes** page 49

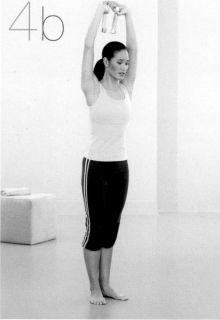

▲ **Salutes** page 49

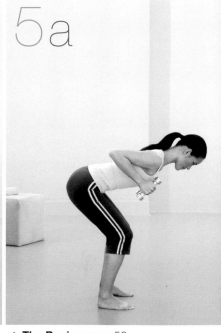

▲ **The Boxing** page 50

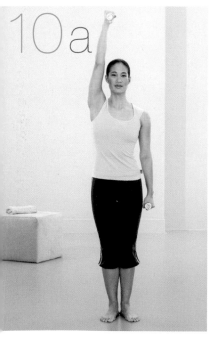

▲ **Side Bend** page 55

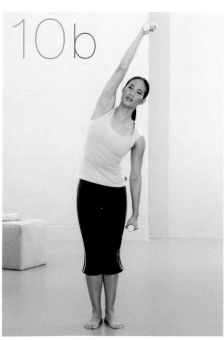

▲ **Side Bend** page 55

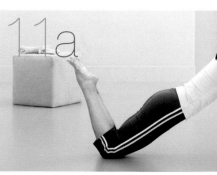

▲ **Push-ups**
page 56

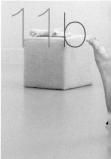

▲ **Push-ups** page 5

>> **from the top down** extras

It's easy to feel the pull of resistance when you do this routine, which involves working with weights. As an experiment, once you've performed this programme, do a run-through without any weights but force your muscles to behave as though you were still holding them. This is the essence of internal resistance.

>> **Checklist**

Remember to move from your centre. Although these exercises appear to be for the limbs, they are just as much for your core.

• Did you work within your 'frame' – keeping your arms within your peripheral vision?

• Have you worked with internal resistance throughout each movement of the programme?

• Can you feel how the lower body must stabilize in order to mobilize the upper body?

• During the Front Curls, as in all Pilates standing positions, were you positioned very slightly forwards on your feet as though you were 'leaning into the wind'?

• For the Side Curls, were you able to keep pressing the shoulders down using the muscles of your back?

• Are you able to maintain your vertical alignment during the Zip-ups and Salutes so that your spine does not waver?

• Some of the hand-weight exercises are done in parallel. Can you keep your legs aligned so that your feet, knees and hips are all pointing straight forwards?

• Did you remember to keep some weight on the outside foot while side-bending away from that leg?

• The Lunges can be tricky with respect to timing. Did you co-ordinate the return of the leg and the lowering of the arms so that they end simultaneously?

>> Modify/Adjust

Hand weights add another element to your workout. Be sure to work deliberately and carefully through each section.

• Change the angle of the limbs to reduce your range of motion for the arm-weight exercises to make them slightly easier.

• Alter your position if you must, bending the knees less deeply during the flat-back exercises to reduce the intensity.

• Remember to decrease your weights or eliminate them as necessary if undue strain occurs.

>> Challenge

You can make an exercise harder by increasing your repetitions or slowing down your tempo. You can also focus on the exacting detail of each move for a real challenge.

• Learn to hold your body still regardless of the movement of the circling arms while you perform the Baby Circles.

• Practise the Lunges focusing on the drag-in to work on activating that hard-to-reach area, the inner thighs.

• Try to increase the weights by 0.5–1kg (1–2lb) as you improve. Don't go above 1.8–2.25kg (4–5lb) total.

>> Trainer tips

Work the transitions. Make your connecting movements every bit as important as the main exercises.

• Be sure your breathing is focused and targeted. Always inhale to prepare and exhale as you execute a movement.

• Work with the joint. Be careful not to lock or jam your elbows or knees as you move through the series. Remember that your muscles move your bones, not the other way around.

• As you perform your hand-weight series, aim to keep your wrists in an elongated hold. Extending the wrists long provides increased stability to your forearms as opposed to bending or cocking the wrists and weakening your grip on the weights.

15 minute

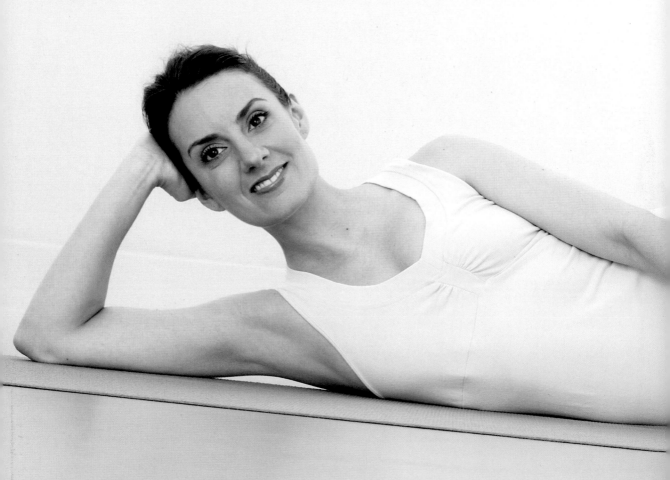

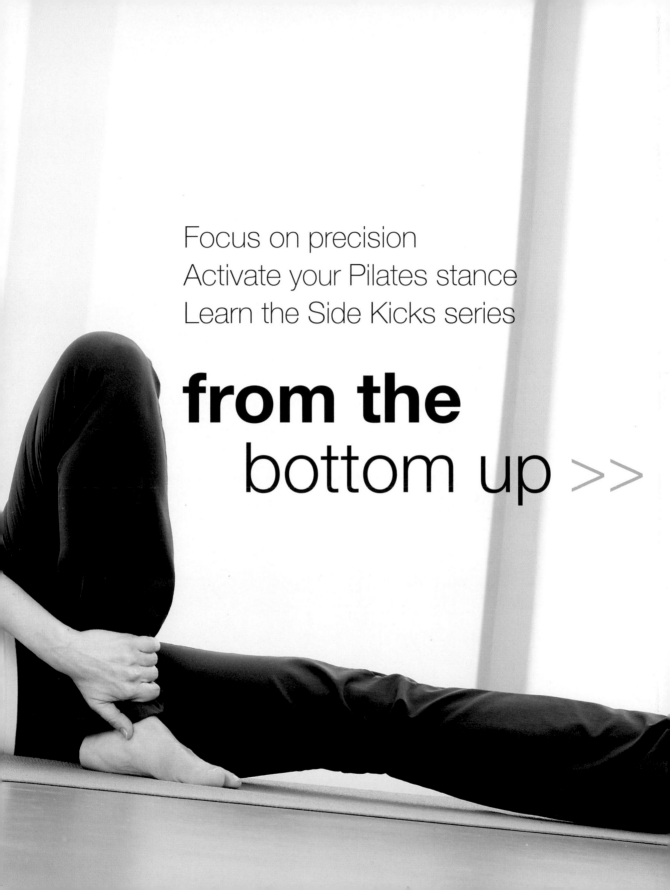

Focus on precision
Activate your Pilates stance
Learn the Side Kicks series

from the
bottom up >>

>> **from the** bottom up

This programme begins with some preparatory moves and concludes, as does the last programme, with an upright exercise. It will build stamina and emphasize centring. By now you should begin to feel comfortable executing the exercises without sacrificing either your form or the key concepts.

We begin with two exercises of my own design that use the Pilates stance with the legs extended in a non-weight-bearing position. We then move into a side-lying position for the classic Pilates Side Kicks series. Transferring to a seated position, we'll perform a modified Teaser – the 'poster pose' for Pilates exercises. This version is meant to work your abdominals and challenge your control as you descend from the pose. The routine rounds off with some moves taken from the Pilates equipment, namely the Hug and the Standing Arm Circles. In between, you'll find the Mermaid, an exercise which totally embodies the grace and fluidity of the Pilates system.

Starting and finishing
As you sit on the mat at the start with your legs outstretched, forget about the muscles you are planning to work. Begin by activating all the other muscle groups. Sit with tall posture, a lifted waist and a long neck. As you adjust your body to get ready for Pilates stance, take note of how much should be done in preparation for each exercise.

The final exercise, Arm Circles, is done standing in this programme. Although Arm Circles are traditionally performed on Pilates equipment, this variation gets you off the floor and ready for real life.

Transitions
Here, the links between exercises are more complex than before. Approach the Side Kicks Preparation as a position of stability. If you are

>> **secrets of** success

- **Pilates stance** is initiated from the buttocks. To do this correctly when sitting, draw the buttock muscles together. You should then rise slightly off your mat.

- **During the up/down** in the Side Kicks, pay special attention to the tempo changes. The leg travels up loosely but lowers down with increasing resistance.

- **The Mermaid** is a lengthening exercise, not a bending one. Be sure not to collapse into your waist. Instead pull up out of your bottom half as though you were being lifted up by your upper arm.

properly positioned you should require very little adjusting. As you progress, resist relaxing your leg in between moves, but stay controlled, using the end of one exercise as the start of the next. When you transfer onto the stomach for the Beats, use minimal movement. Although the Teaser's focus is in its second half, don't ignore your form in the first. This programme synthesizes all you have learned.

The Mermaid is a classic Pilates exercise. By anchoring the lower half of the body, the upper half is free to lengthen and stretch.

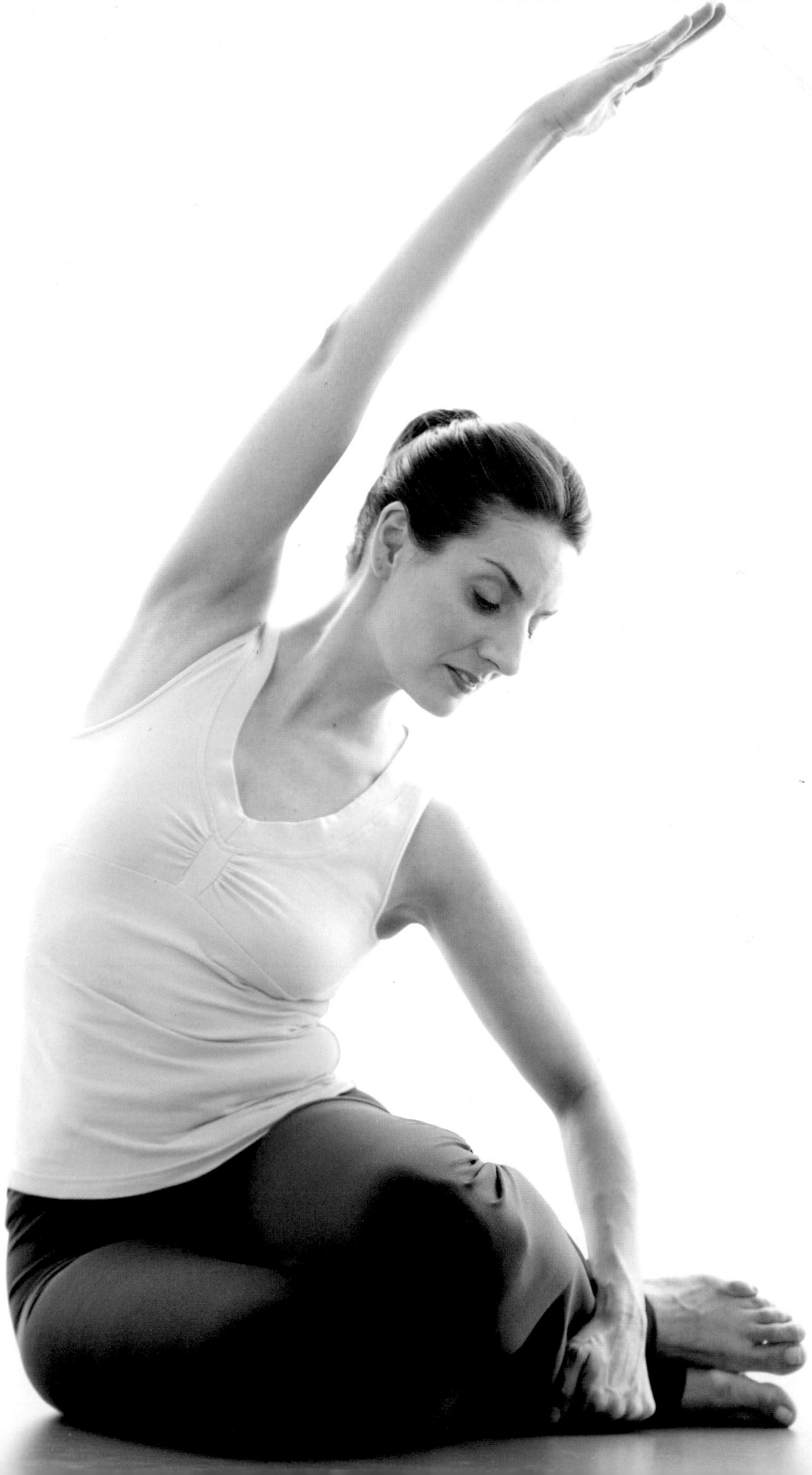

>> pilates stance 1 & 2

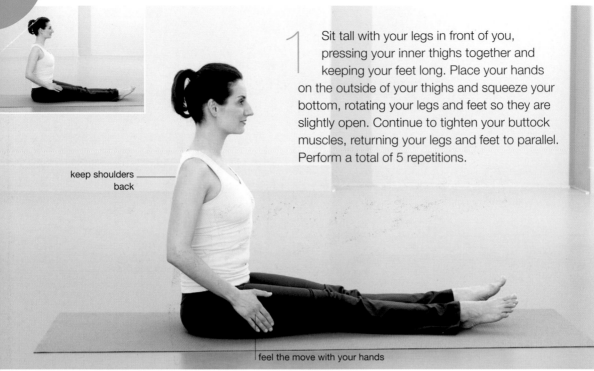

1 Sit tall with your legs in front of you, pressing your inner thighs together and keeping your feet long. Place your hands on the outside of your thighs and squeeze your bottom, rotating your legs and feet so they are slightly open. Continue to tighten your buttock muscles, returning your legs and feet to parallel. Perform a total of 5 repetitions.

keep shoulders back

feel the move with your hands

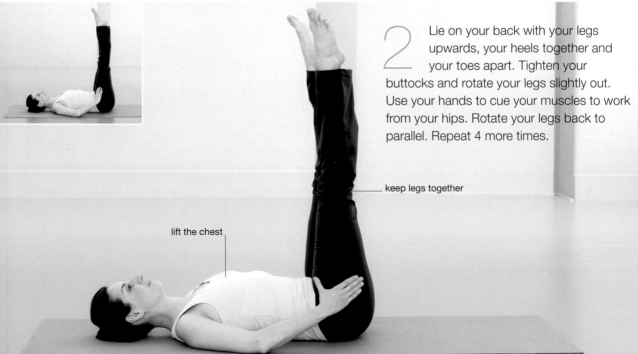

2 Lie on your back with your legs upwards, your heels together and your toes apart. Tighten your buttocks and rotate your legs slightly out. Use your hands to cue your muscles to work from your hips. Rotate your legs back to parallel. Repeat 4 more times.

keep legs together

lift the chest

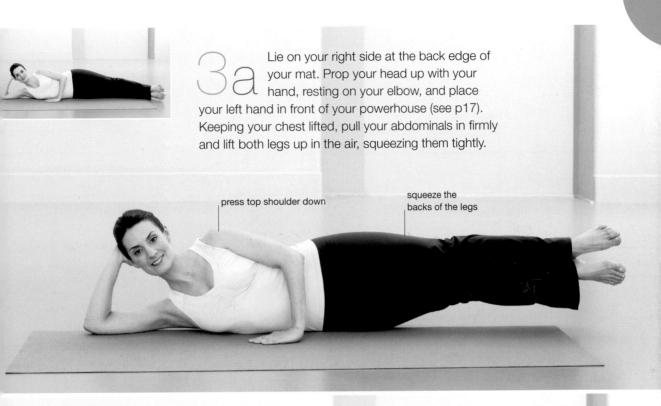

3a Lie on your right side at the back edge of your mat. Prop your head up with your hand, resting on your elbow, and place your left hand in front of your powerhouse (see p17). Keeping your chest lifted, pull your abdominals in firmly and lift both legs up in the air, squeezing them tightly.

press top shoulder down

squeeze the backs of the legs

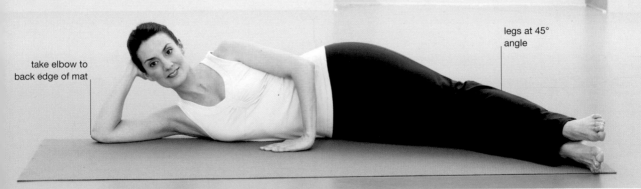

3b Without disrupting your posture, carry your legs forwards to the front edge of the mat and lower them with control. You should be at a 45° angle on the mat, with your hips and shoulders stacked one on top of the other.

take elbow to back edge of mat

legs at 45° angle

from the bottom up >>

>> **side kicks front**

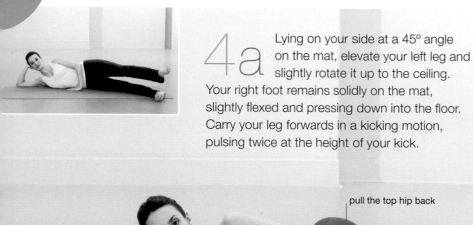

4a Lying on your side at a 45° angle on the mat, elevate your left leg and slightly rotate it up to the ceiling. Your right foot remains solidly on the mat, slightly flexed and pressing down into the floor. Carry your leg forwards in a kicking motion, pulsing twice at the height of your kick.

pull the top hip back

don't rotate the bottom leg

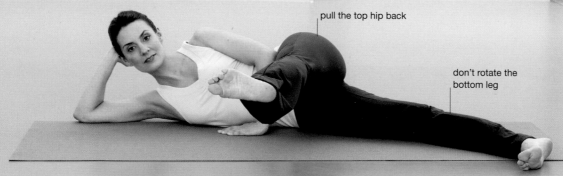

4b Sweep the leg down and back behind the body, tightening the buttock muscles. Keep the upper body still and strong. Repeat a total of 6 times, perfecting your form each time. Bring the leg back to its starting position.

don't lean forwards

keep hips stacked

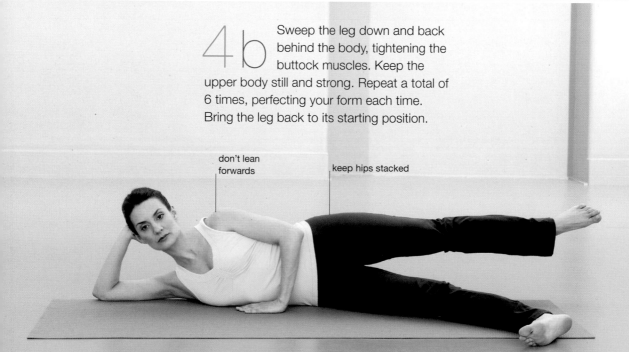

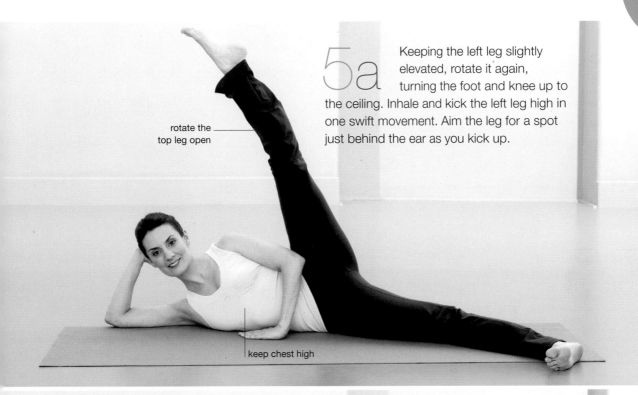

5a Keeping the left leg slightly elevated, rotate it again, turning the foot and knee up to the ceiling. Inhale and kick the left leg high in one swift movement. Aim the leg for a spot just behind the ear as you kick up.

rotate the top leg open

keep chest high

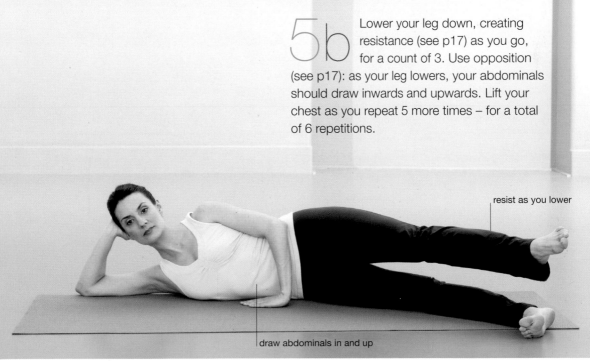

5b Lower your leg down, creating resistance (see p17) as you go, for a count of 3. Use opposition (see p17): as your leg lowers, your abdominals should draw inwards and upwards. Lift your chest as you repeat 5 more times – for a total of 6 repetitions.

resist as you lower

draw abdominals in and up

>> **side kicks circles**

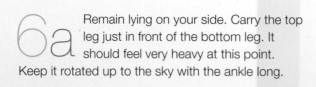

6a Remain lying on your side. Carry the top leg just in front of the bottom leg. It should feel very heavy at this point. Keep it rotated up to the sky with the ankle long.

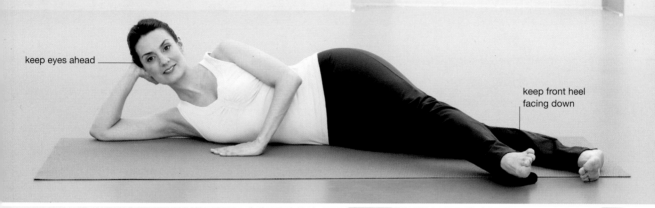

keep eyes ahead

keep front heel facing down

6b Draw 10 tiny circles with the leg in the air without shaking your body. Pause briefly. Switch immediately, taking the left leg back and reversing the circles. Keep the circles tiny and emphasize the downwards portion of the circle. Repeat 10 circles and pause before resting the left leg on the right.

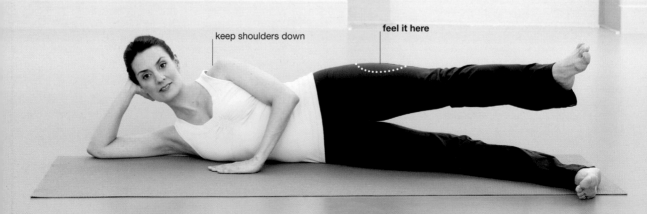

keep shoulders down

feel it here

7a Remain lying on your right side. Cross the left leg in front of the right leg and take hold of the ankle. Place the left foot flat on the floor with the knee and foot pointing down towards the bottom foot. Now, flex the right foot and lift the entire right leg just above the mat.

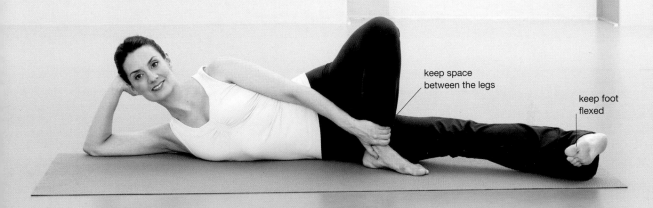

keep space between the legs

keep foot flexed

7b Without hunching or collapsing, raise the right leg to its highest point and lower it back to above the mat. Repeat 7 more times for a total of 8 repetitions. On the last repetition, remain at the highest point and perfect the position by lengthening, straightening and rotating just a little bit more. Finally, lower the leg with control.

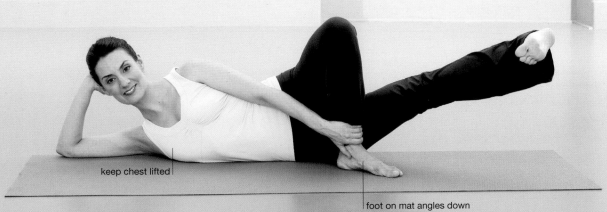

keep chest lifted

foot on mat angles down

>> **side kicks bicycle**

8a Lie with the legs together at a 45° angle in front of you. Raise the left leg slightly. Swing it out in front of the body without hunching or rounding the back. Create opposition by pulling back, or retracting, the left hip behind you slightly. Bend the left knee in towards the shoulder.

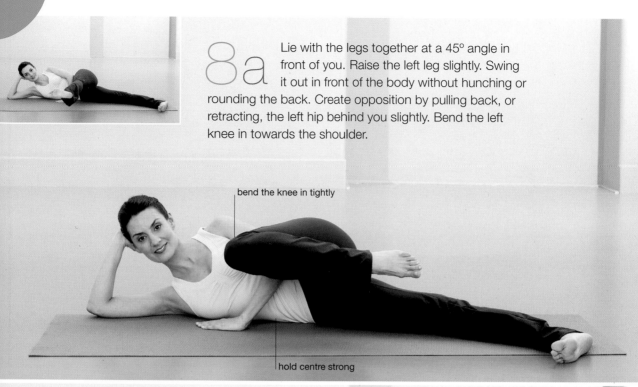

bend the knee in tightly

hold centre strong

8b Sweep the left knee down next to the right knee before extending it behind you. Pull the waist up in opposition to the leg reaching down. Repeat 2 more times and then return the leg to its start position. Reverse direction for 3 more repetitions.

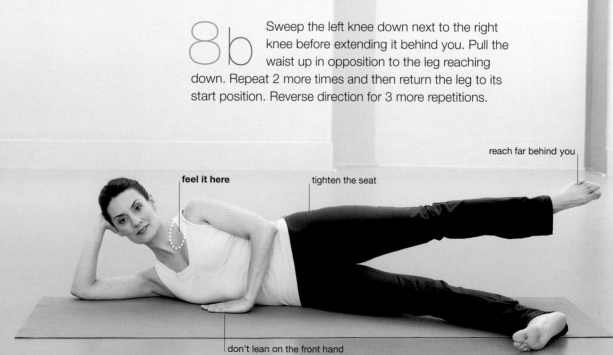

reach far behind you

feel it here

tighten the seat

don't lean on the front hand

9a Transition onto your stomach, then lie face down on your mat. Place your hands under your forehead and stretch your legs out. Tighten your abdominals and elevate both legs slightly. Keep your shoulders pulling back and down as you open your legs and start to beat them together.

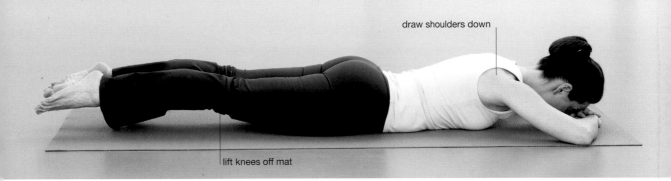

draw shoulders down

lift knees off mat

9b Breathing naturally, continue beating briskly for 20 counts. Beat the legs from the upper inner thighs and keep the knees straight. Pause at the end to lengthen the legs, tighten the abs and soften the neck and shoulders, before lowering the legs with control. Roll over onto the other side and repeat the Side Kicks series (Steps 3a–8b) with the opposite leg.

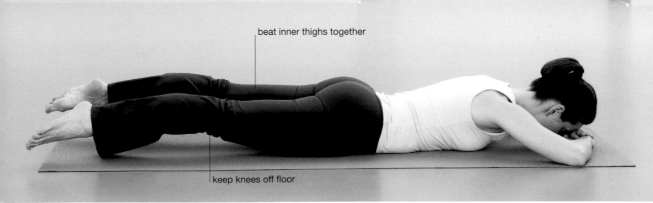

beat inner thighs together

keep knees off floor

>> **the teaser**

10a Transition onto your back and bring your knees into your chest as you reach your arms overhead.

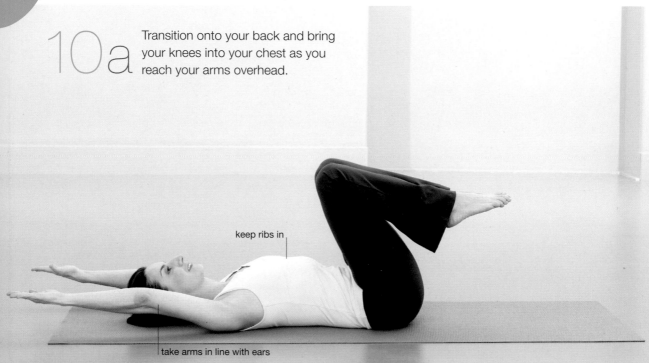

keep ribs in

take arms in line with ears

10b In one count, sweep your body up to sitting, balancing with your legs at 90°, arms reaching forwards, abs deeply scooped, chest open. With control, curl your tail under you, laying your spine onto the mat. Fold your knees in, arms overhead to repeat. Perform 5 repetitions.

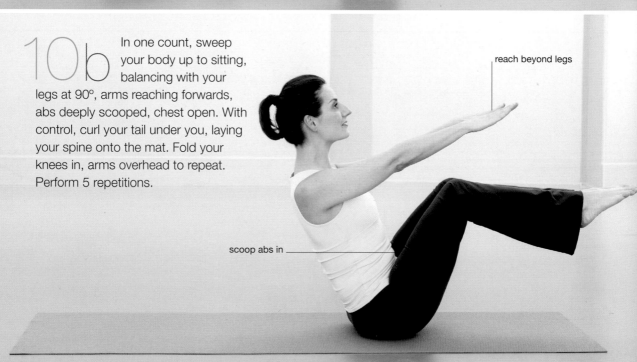

reach beyond legs

scoop abs in

>> **the hug**

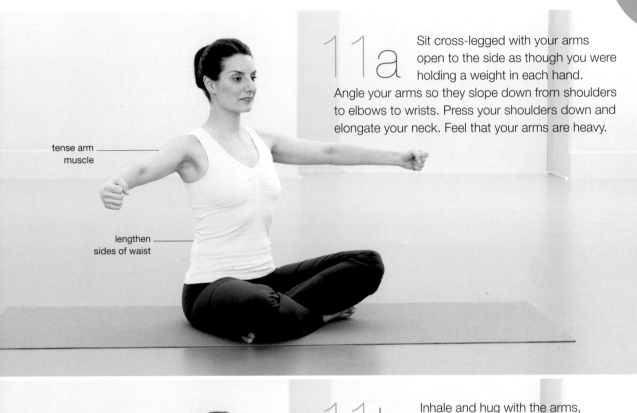

11a

Sit cross-legged with your arms open to the side as though you were holding a weight in each hand. Angle your arms so they slope down from shoulders to elbows to wrists. Press your shoulders down and elongate your neck. Feel that your arms are heavy.

tense arm muscle

lengthen sides of waist

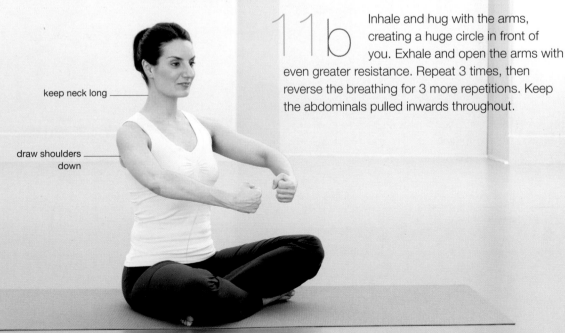

11b

Inhale and hug with the arms, creating a huge circle in front of you. Exhale and open the arms with even greater resistance. Repeat 3 times, then reverse the breathing for 3 more repetitions. Keep the abdominals pulled inwards throughout.

keep neck long

draw shoulders down

>> **the mermaid**

12a Sit to the right side of your legs with your knees, shins and ankles stacked on your left. Reach your left hand underneath your bottom ankle and hook onto it, holding firmly. Sweep your free right arm up overhead and inhale to prepare.

lengthen waist _____

hold the bottom
ankle firmly

12b Bend lightly over the legs, exhaling as you stretch the right side. Reach the arm and body higher up as you return to upright. Repeat 2 more times, pausing at the end, lifting the waist and pulling the shoulders down. Swing the legs to the other side for 3 more repetitions.

_____ reach up and over

_____ open elbow out

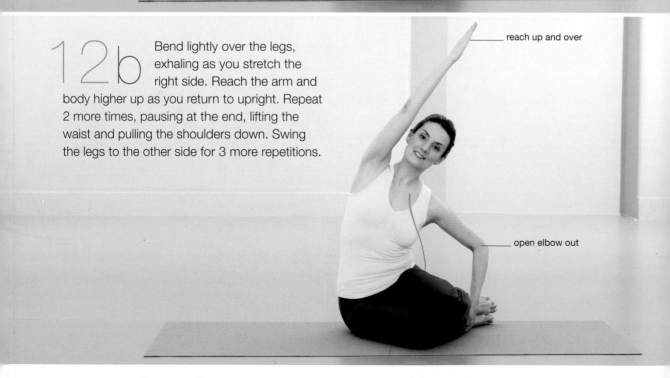

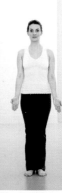

13a Stand in Pilates stance (see p17). Shift your weight slightly forwards. Hold your arms by your thighs with your palms facing forwards. Inhale, then exhale and raise your arms straight up to the sky.

13b Flip the palms outwards and circle the arms down, exerting pressure as though the air were thick. Repeat 2 more times, then reverse the breath, inhaling on the raise and exhaling on the lower, for another 3 repetitions.

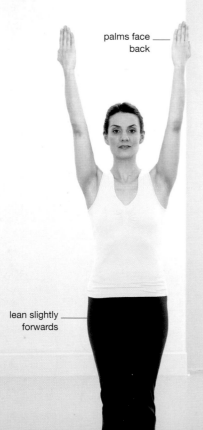

palms face back

lean slightly forwards

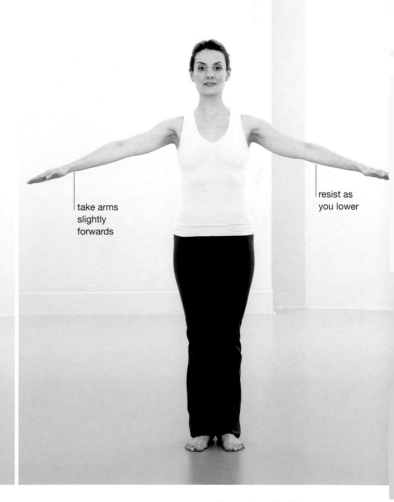

take arms slightly forwards

resist as you lower

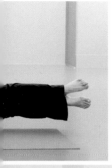

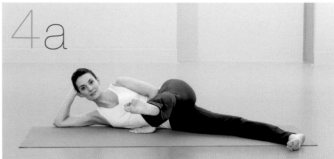

4a

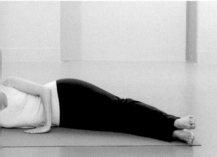

▲ **Side Kicks Front** page 72

...ation page 71

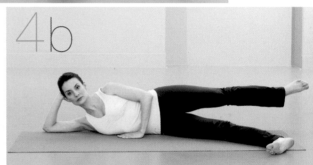

4b

▲ **Side Kicks Front** page 72

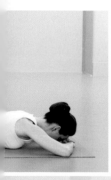

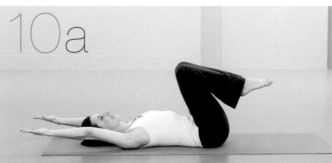

10a

▲ **The Teaser** page 78

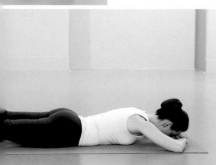

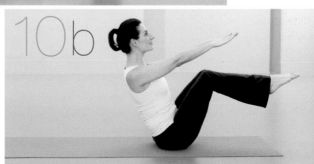

10b

page 77

▲ **The Teaser** page 78

summary from the bottom up

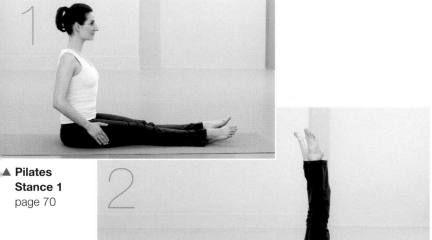

▲ **Pilates
Stance 1**
page 70

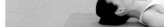

▲ **Pilates Stance 2** page 70

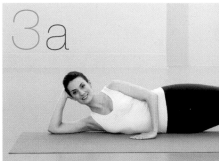

▲ **Side Kicks
Preparation**
page 71

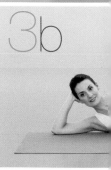

▲ **Side Kicks Prepa**

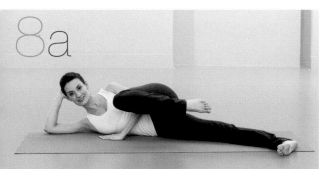

▲ **Side Kicks
Bicycle**
page 76

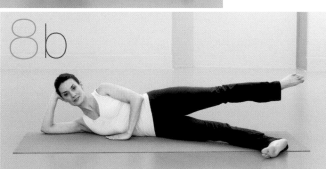

▲ **Side Kicks Bicycle** page 76

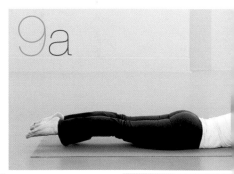

▲ **Beats on
Stomach**
page 77

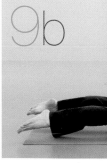

▲ **Beats on Stomac**

from the bottom up >>

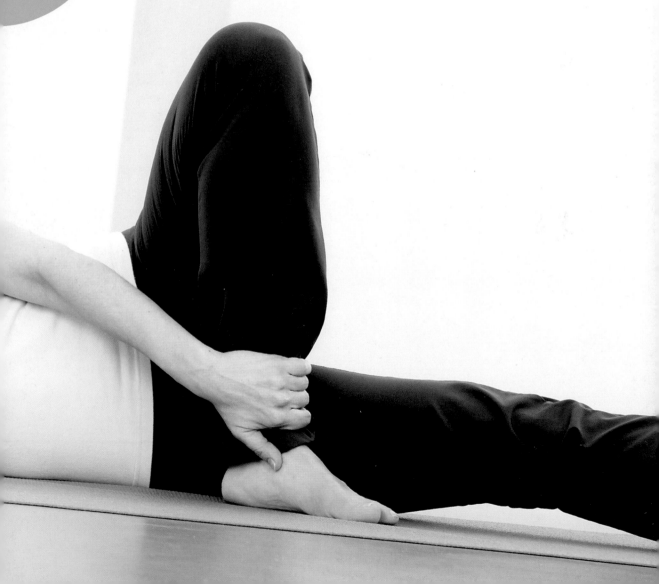

15 minute **summary**

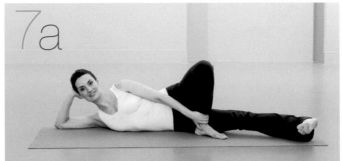

7a

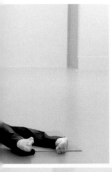

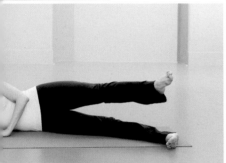

▲ Side Kicks
Inner-thigh
Lifts
page 75

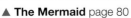
page 74

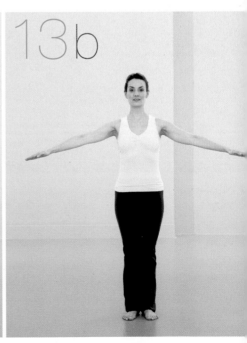

7b

▲ **Side Kicks Inner-thigh Lifts** page 75

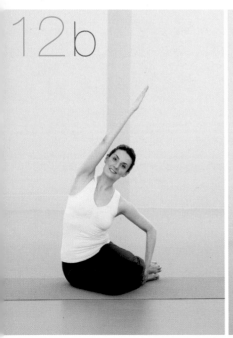

12b

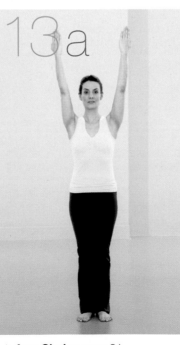

13a

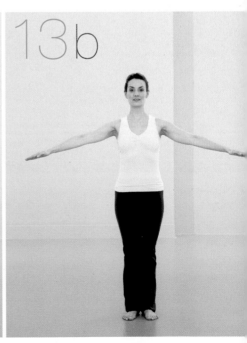

13b

▲ **The Mermaid** page 80

▲ **Arm Circles** page 81

▲ **Arm Circles** page 81

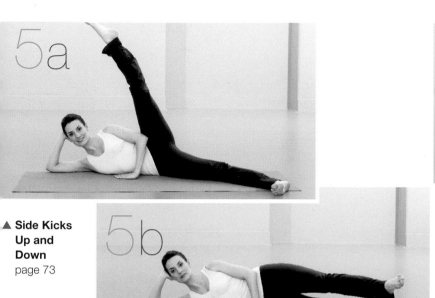

5a

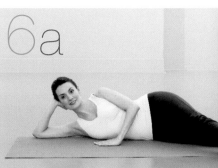

6a

▲ **Side Kicks Circles** page 74

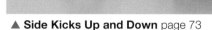

▲ **Side Kicks Up and Down** page 73

5b

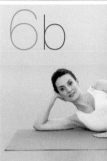

6b

▲ **Side Kicks Up and Down** page 73

▲ **Side Kicks Circle**

▲ **Side Kicks Up and Down** page 73

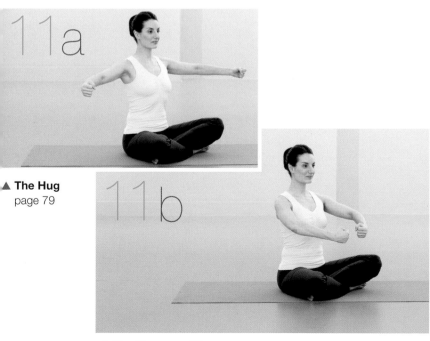

11a

▲ **The Hug** page 79

11b

▲ **The Hug** page 79

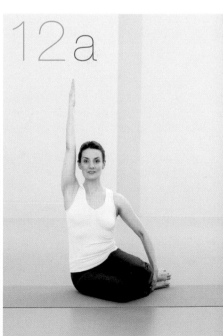

12a

▲ **The Mermaid** page 80

>> **from the bottom up** extras

Remember the old-style workouts like calisthenics? The Bottom Up programme looks eerily similar. The critical difference is precision and form. Focus on controlling your movements rather than hurling your body around. You'll accomplish both form and function at the same time.

>> **Checklist**

Every portion of every exercise is equally important. If you believe you've mastered a move, look again.

• Did you work with opposition, lengthening the torso against the limbs and vice versa?

• Have you focused on what the top half of the body is doing during this lower-body series?

• Can you incorporate your Pilates stance exercises into the rest of the mat exercises, even when the legs are in the air?

• During Pilates Stance 2, could you feel with your hands that your rotation muscles were pulling the legs into position?

• The Side Kicks focus so heavily on the lower body that people forget their upper bodies. Did you keep your chest lifted and shoulders down throughout?

• For the Side Kicks Front and the Side Kicks Circles, did you maintain your torso alignment without rolling onto the front hand when the leg travelled behind you?

• When you are performing the Beats on Stomach, can you actively draw your shoulder blades down and together in order to avoid hunching and to keep the chest open?

>> Modify/Adjust

Remember, to decrease the intensity you must draw your limbs closer to your centre. If you must bend them, go ahead.

• Change the leg position into parallel if the rotation of the hips is too intense during the Side Kicks.

• Alter your position to separate your legs for the Mermaid, instead of allowing your shins to rest against one another.

>> Challenge

Experiment with your own positions. A slight pivot or angle change can alter an exercise dramatically.

• Learn to anchor the bottom leg while you are performing the Side Kicks series to increase your stability.

• Attempt to perform the Teaser with legs extended at a 45° angle as you rise up and as you lower.

• Try to add light ankle weights to the Side Kicks if the exercises become too easy.

• Switch the hand on the mat to behind the head for the Side Kicks series. Keep your elbow pointing to the sky.

>> Trainer tips

Use your eyes to position your legs where they look the best, then work from there, making sure the muscles look taut and shapely.

• I constructed the Pilates stance exercises to provide a support system for much of the work we do in the Pilates method, so practise those regularly. Remember to initiate from your hips.

• This Teaser version is my own and is meant to eliminate self-doubt and to work the core. Remember to focus on the descent.

• It's a good idea to trick your body every now and then by starting on a different side. If you typically begin your leg series on the right, alternate on certain days to begin with the left. Similarly, if you find that you sit cross-legged with the right leg on top all the time, make a change every now and then.

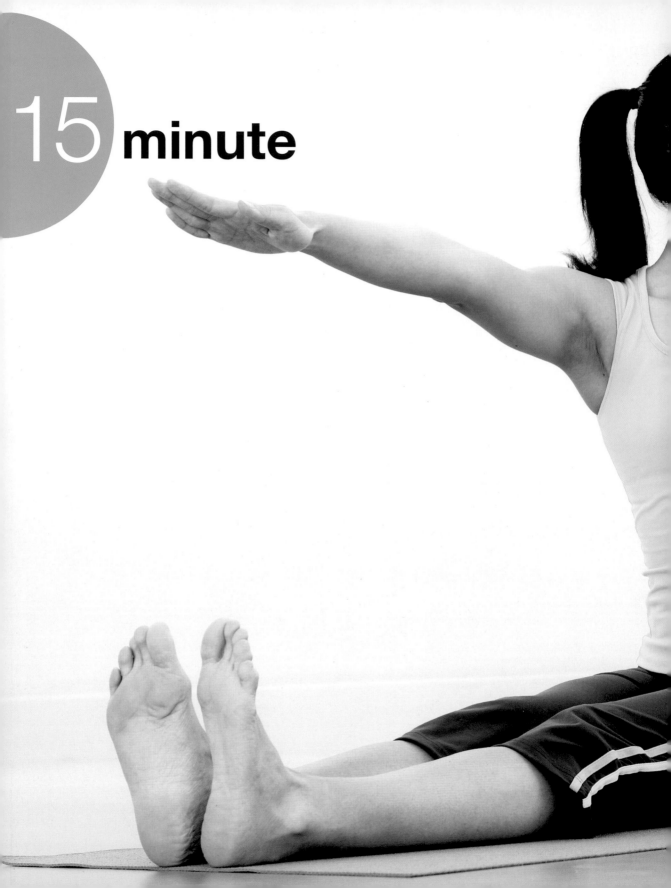

15 minute

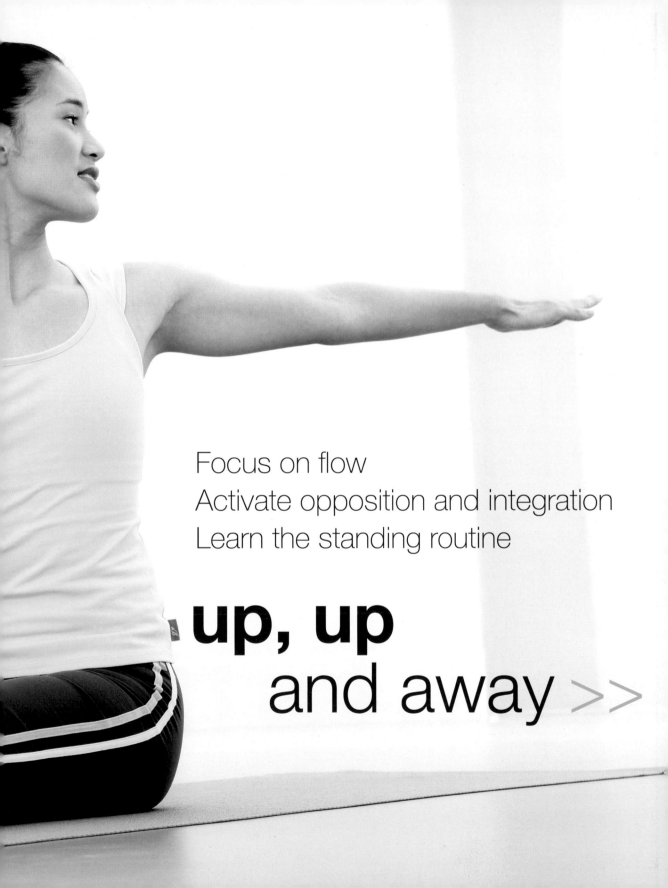

Focus on flow
Activate opposition and integration
Learn the standing routine

up, up
and away >>

>> **up, up and** away

This last programme establishes the muscle memory you will need to set you up for everyday life. We often need to bend, twist, lean and reach – all moves you will perform here. Your ultimate goal is to subconsciously incorporate your Pilates practice into every waking moment for a stronger, safer body.

The programme begins with two seated exercises that help with those all-too-common neck misalignments. We follow these with a challenging variation of the Hundred and some classic Pilates Rowing exercises. Then it's onto our knees for some more classic exercises that reinforce our use of internal resistance. When we come up to standing, we will perform some historical Pilates exercises to strengthen our lower limbs.

Starting and finishing

As you begin the Neck Strengthener, take a minute to fix your posture. Your neck is an extension of your spine and it will be impossible to align your neck if your spine is rounded over. Take note of the top of your head where it begins to slope downwards in a curve. This is the crown of the head. As you sit, stand, kneel or lie, you should always be reaching the crown of the head up and away from you.

You end with the Sides Splits – a functional exercise group. By training your body to engage your core during these dynamic moving exercises, you are preparing for the unexpected movements that you will encounter in real life. Here, focus on your waistline pulling up and away from your legs as you drag the legs together each time.

Transitions

Transfer in controlled, neat movements from the opening neck exercises to the seated movements. To transition to kneeling, tuck your knees into your

>> **secrets** of success

- **Many find the Chest Expansion** rather subtle. Remember to activate your powerhouse (see p17) and pull your arms behind you as you turn your head.

- **When you kneel** during the Thigh Stretch, tighten all your muscles from top to tail. You should lock your body as though it were a piece of steel.

- **The Footwork series** comprises historical Pilates moves. These squat-like movements require full-body integration.

body and then bring them underneath you, raising up your torso as you do so. When it's time to stand, you need only to place your hands on the mat, tuck your toes underneath you and roll up to standing. As you move from one exercise in the Footwork series to the next, pay special attention to the alignment of your upper body. No matter how you get there, using symmetrical efficient movement without expending excess energy should be your goal.

Up, Up and Away will reinforce the total-body integration of Pilates. Prepare your body for everyday life by taking the philosophy of Pilates with you everywhere.

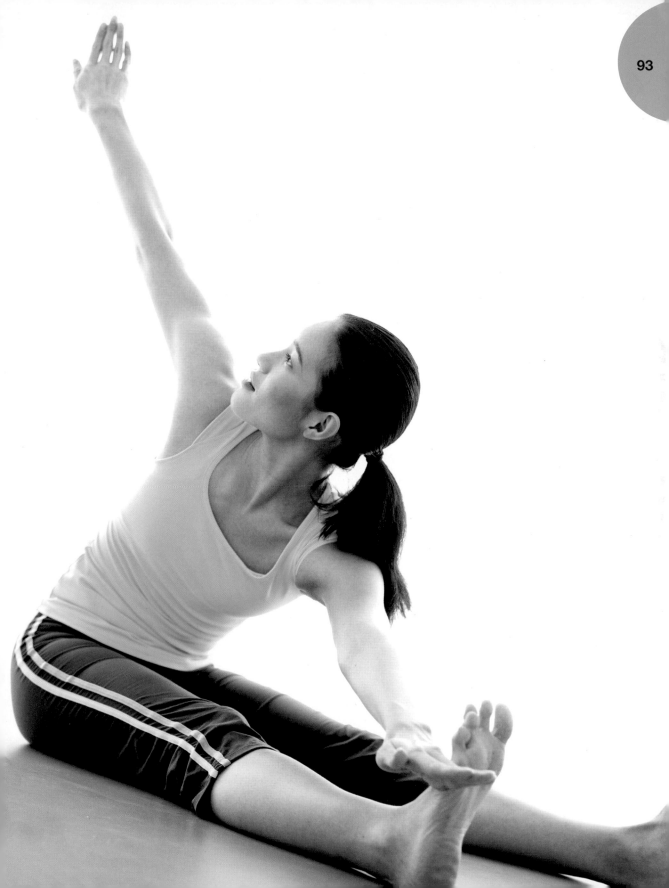

>> **neck press/shoulder roll**

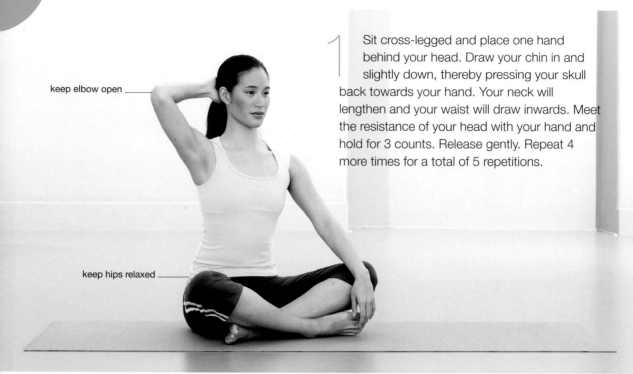

keep elbow open

keep hips relaxed

1 Sit cross-legged and place one hand behind your head. Draw your chin in and slightly down, thereby pressing your skull back towards your hand. Your neck will lengthen and your waist will draw inwards. Meet the resistance of your head with your hand and hold for 3 counts. Release gently. Repeat 4 more times for a total of 5 repetitions.

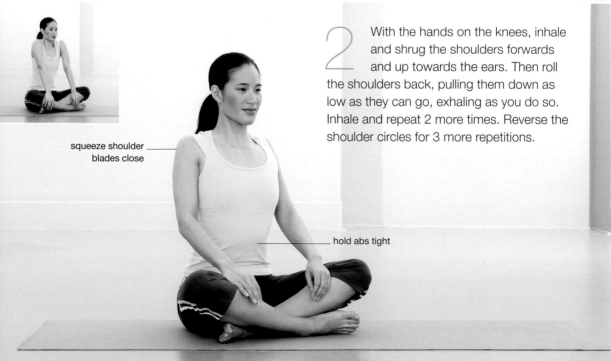

squeeze shoulder blades close

hold abs tight

2 With the hands on the knees, inhale and shrug the shoulders forwards and up towards the ears. Then roll the shoulders back, pulling them down as low as they can go, exhaling as you do so. Inhale and repeat 2 more times. Reverse the shoulder circles for 3 more repetitions.

>> **the hundred**

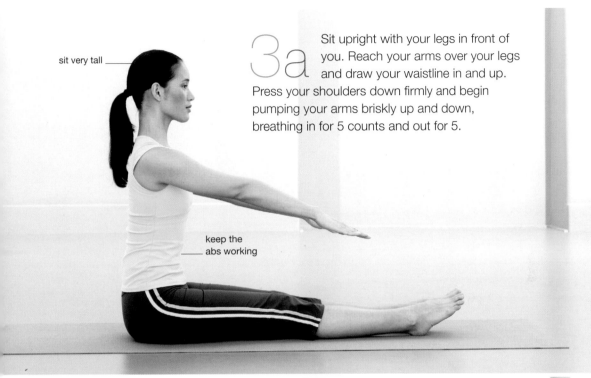

sit very tall

keep the
abs working

3a Sit upright with your legs in front of you. Reach your arms over your legs and draw your waistline in and up. Press your shoulders down firmly and begin pumping your arms briskly up and down, breathing in for 5 counts and out for 5.

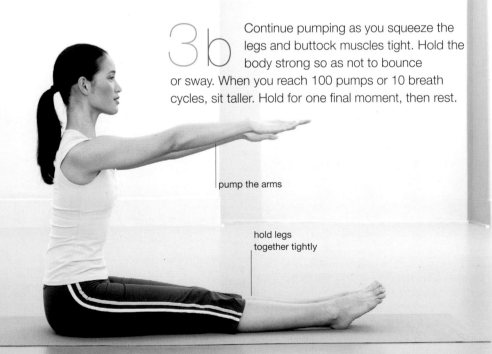

pump the arms

hold legs
together tightly

3b Continue pumping as you squeeze the legs and buttock muscles tight. Hold the body strong so as not to bounce or sway. When you reach 100 pumps or 10 breath cycles, sit taller. Hold for one final moment, then rest.

>> **rowing 1**

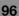

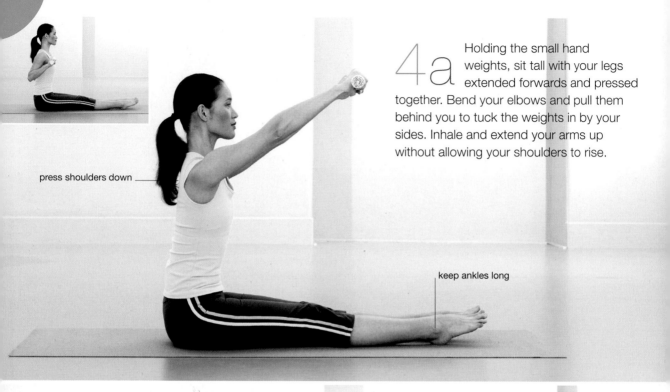

press shoulders down

keep ankles long

4a Holding the small hand weights, sit tall with your legs extended forwards and pressed together. Bend your elbows and pull them behind you to tuck the weights in by your sides. Inhale and extend your arms up without allowing your shoulders to rise.

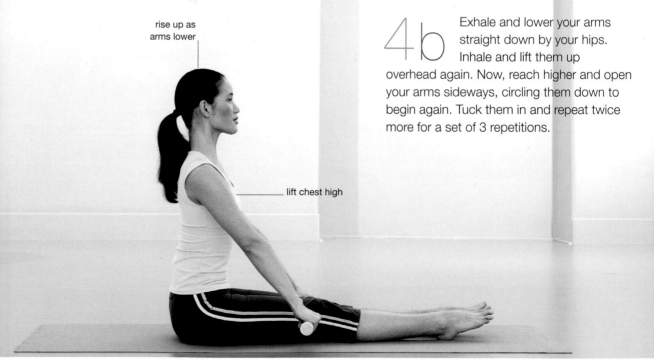

rise up as
arms lower

lift chest high

4b Exhale and lower your arms straight down by your hips. Inhale and lift them up overhead again. Now, reach higher and open your arms sideways, circling them down to begin again. Tuck them in and repeat twice more for a set of 3 repetitions.

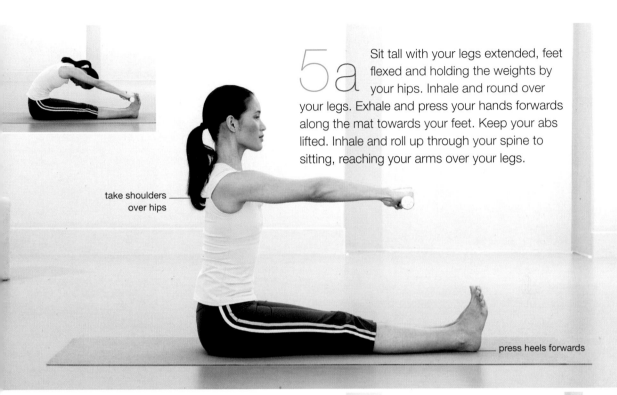

5a Sit tall with your legs extended, feet flexed and holding the weights by your hips. Inhale and round over your legs. Exhale and press your hands forwards along the mat towards your feet. Keep your abs lifted. Inhale and roll up through your spine to sitting, reaching your arms over your legs.

take shoulders over hips

press heels forwards

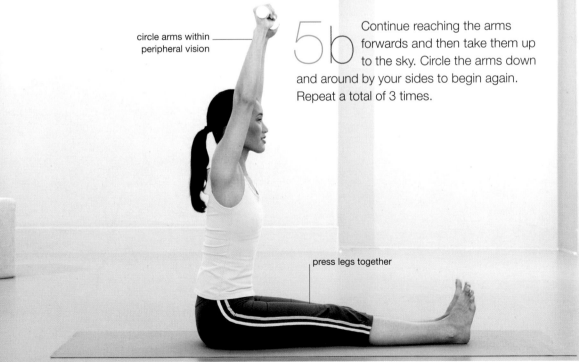

circle arms within peripheral vision

5b Continue reaching the arms forwards and then take them up to the sky. Circle the arms down and around by your sides to begin again. Repeat a total of 3 times.

press legs together

>> spine twist

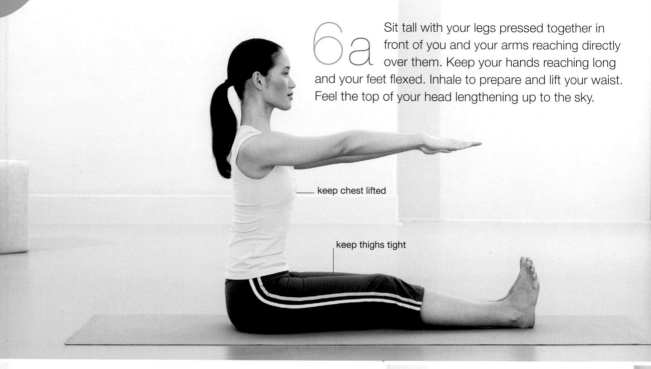

6a Sit tall with your legs pressed together in front of you and your arms reaching directly over them. Keep your hands reaching long and your feet flexed. Inhale to prepare and lift your waist. Feel the top of your head lengthening up to the sky.

keep chest lifted

keep thighs tight

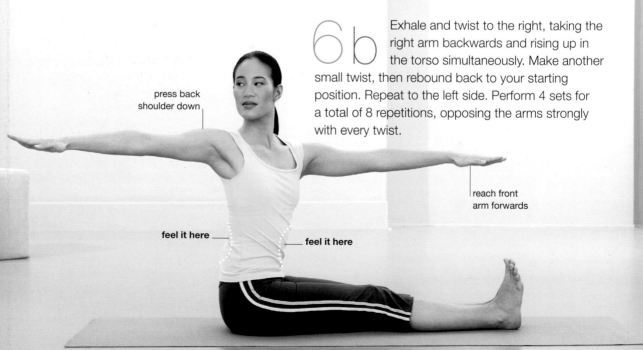

6b Exhale and twist to the right, taking the right arm backwards and rising up in the torso simultaneously. Make another small twist, then rebound back to your starting position. Repeat to the left side. Perform 4 sets for a total of 8 repetitions, opposing the arms strongly with every twist.

press back shoulder down

reach front arm forwards

feel it here

feel it here

>> the saw

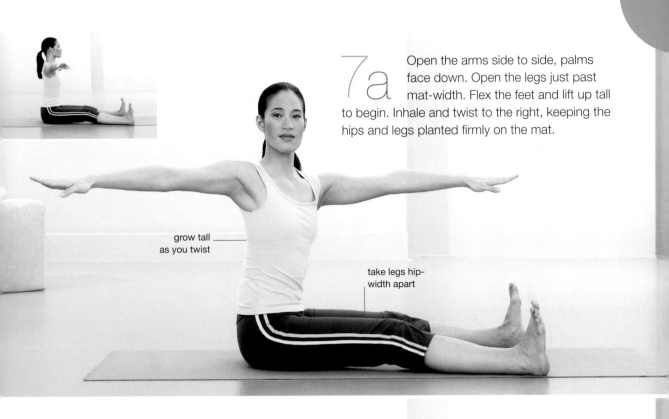

7a

Open the arms side to side, palms face down. Open the legs just past mat-width. Flex the feet and lift up tall to begin. Inhale and twist to the right, keeping the hips and legs planted firmly on the mat.

grow tall
as you twist

take legs hip-
width apart

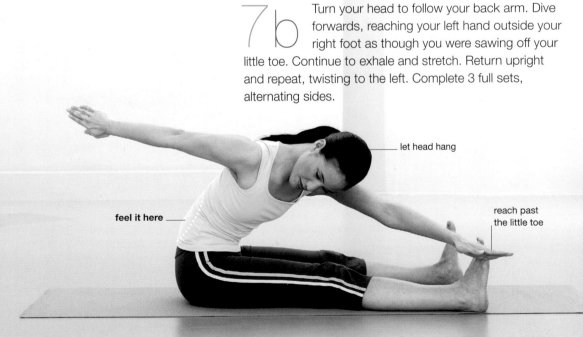

7b

Turn your head to follow your back arm. Dive forwards, reaching your left hand outside your right foot as though you were sawing off your little toe. Continue to exhale and stretch. Return upright and repeat, twisting to the left. Complete 3 full sets, alternating sides.

let head hang

feel it here

reach past
the little toe

>> lotus

8a Take your weights and kneel upright on your mat with your knees comfortably apart. Your arms extend to the sides of your body with the palms face up. Hold strong in your core and keep your chest lifted.

8b Without disrupting your posture, raise the arms straight up, framing the head and neck in an oval. Lower the arms back down with controlled resistance (see p17). Keep the elbows soft. Repeat for a total of 8 times, exhaling to lift and inhaling to lower.

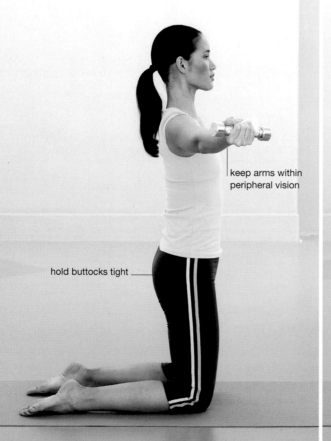

keep arms within peripheral vision

hold buttocks tight

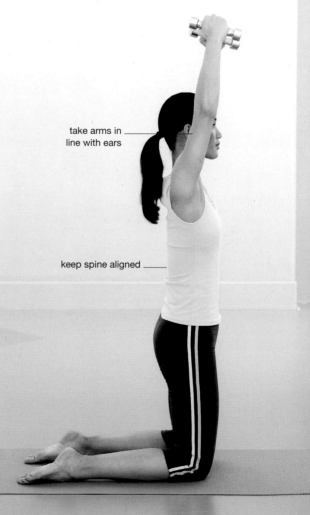

take arms in line with ears

keep spine aligned

>> chest expansion

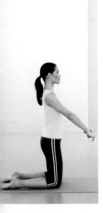

9a Still kneeling upright, hold the weights just in front of you. Tighten the buttocks and pull up in the waist to activate the core. Inhale and sweep the arms behind you with resistance, opening the chest and drawing the shoulder blades together as you go.

9b Keep the arms behind you as you look over the right shoulder and then the left before returning to centre. Exhale and take the arms back in front of you. Repeat 3 more times, alternating the initial direction you turn the head with each set.

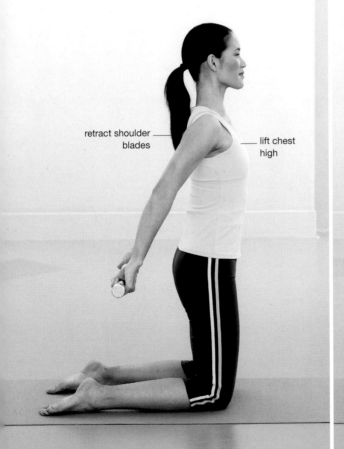

retract shoulder blades

lift chest high

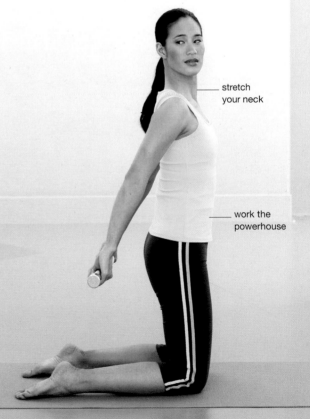

stretch your neck

work the powerhouse

>> thigh stretch

10a Remain on your knees holding the weights with your arms extended directly in front of you just below shoulder-height. Face your palms down and tighten your powerhouse (see p17) to begin. Inhale to prepare.

10b Allow your chin to dip down slightly then hinge back, stretching the fronts of your thighs but not arching your spine. At your lowest point, tighten your buttocks and bring your body back up to start again. Perform a total of 4 repetitions, exhaling each time you rise back up. Put the weights down. Tuck your toes under you to come up to standing.

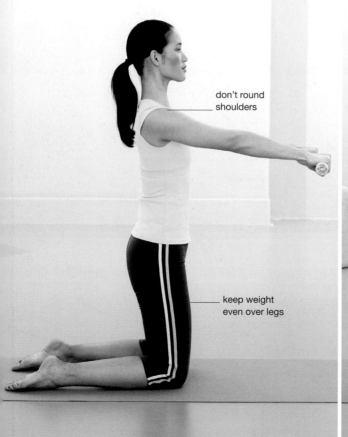

don't round shoulders

keep weight even over legs

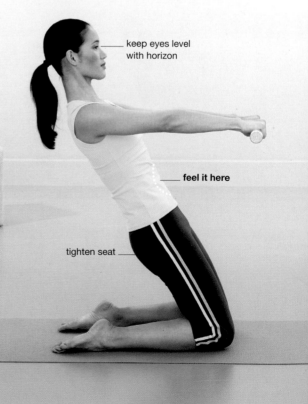

keep eyes level with horizon

feel it here

tighten seat

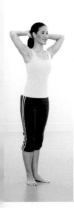

11 Come off your mat and stand up tall in Pilates stance (see p17). Place your hands behind your head, elbows wide. Inhale and bend your knees to lower into a squat. Allow your heels to rise. At the bottom of the squat, press your heels into the floor to rise back up. Perform 6 times, inhaling to lower and exhaling to rise.

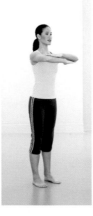

12 Stand with feet parallel, hip-width apart, arms folded in front of you at chest height. Bend your knees as low as you can go, then push your feet into the floor to rise. Repeat for 6 repetitions. Inhale to lower and exhale to rise.

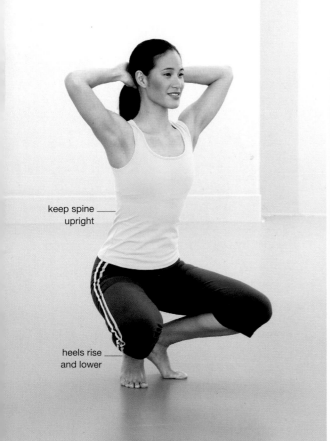

keep spine upright

heels rise and lower

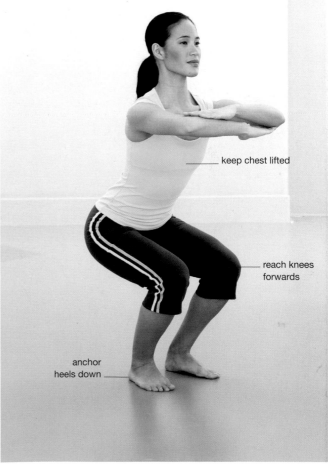

keep chest lifted

reach knees forwards

anchor heels down

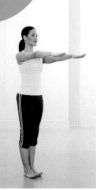

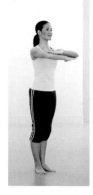

13 Standing with feet together and arms extended in front for stability, curl the toes up and press the rest of the foot firmly down. Pull the abs in, then bend into a squat. Keep the heels down if possible and stay as upright as you can, resisting the urge to bend too far forwards in the spine. Exhale to rise back up with resistance. Don't rush. Repeat a total of 6 times.

14 Return to Pilates stance, with your arms folded in front at chest height. Press down firmly into the floor with the balls of your feet so your heels rise up for 3 counts. Lower down with control. Continue for 6 repetitions, exhaling as you rise and inhaling as you lower.

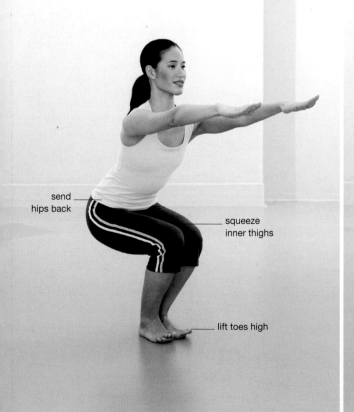

send hips back

squeeze inner thighs

lift toes high

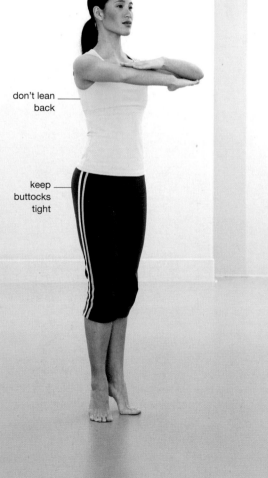

don't lean back

keep buttocks tight

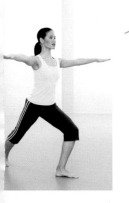

15 Once again, stand in Pilates stance, arms out to your sides. Lunge forwards with your left leg, transferring all your weight onto it. Keep your right leg firmly planted into the floor. Drag your left foot back to the right foot to start again. Inhale to lunge and exhale to pull back 4 times on each leg.

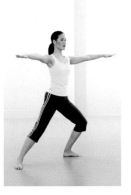

16 Return to Pilates stance, with the arms reaching out to the sides. Lunge sideways with the left leg, then drag the leg home, straightening it as quickly as possible to activate the upper inner thighs. Repeat 3 more times. Repeat with the other leg to the side.

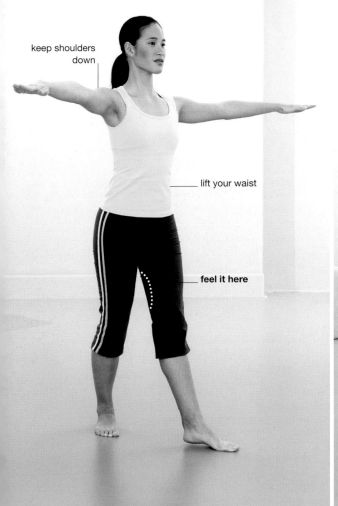

keep shoulders down

lift your waist

feel it here

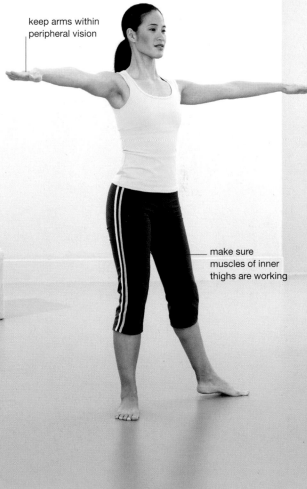

keep arms within peripheral vision

make sure muscles of inner thighs are working

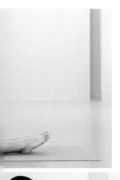

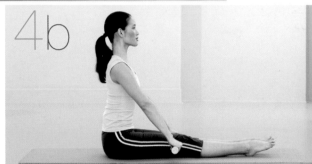

4a

▲ **Rowing 1**
page 96

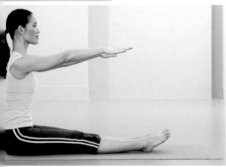

95

4b

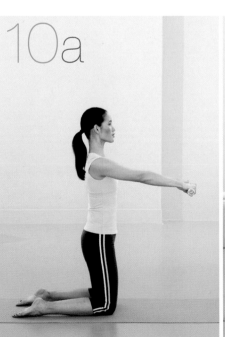

▲ **Rowing 1** page 96

9b

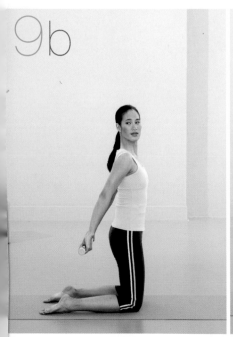

10a

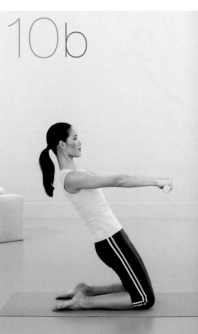

10b

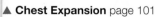

▲ **Chest Expansion** page 101

▲ **Thigh Stretch** page 102

▲ **Thigh Stretch** page 102

summary up, up and away

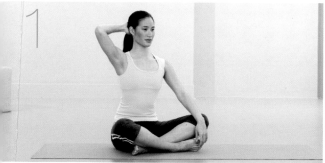

▲ **Neck Press**
page 94

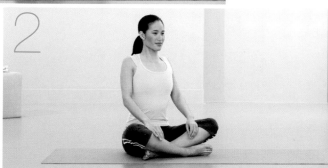

▲ **Shoulder Roll** page 94

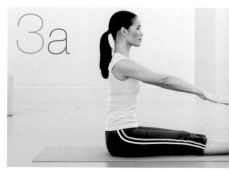

▲ **The Hundred**
page 95

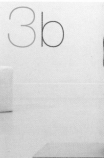

▲ **The Hundred** pag

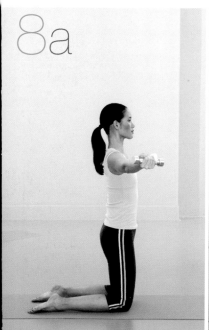

▲ **Lotus** page 100

▲ **Lotus** page 100

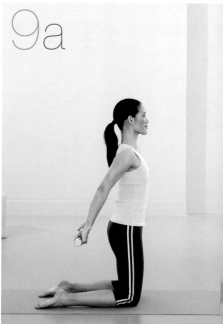

▲ **Chest Expansion** page 101

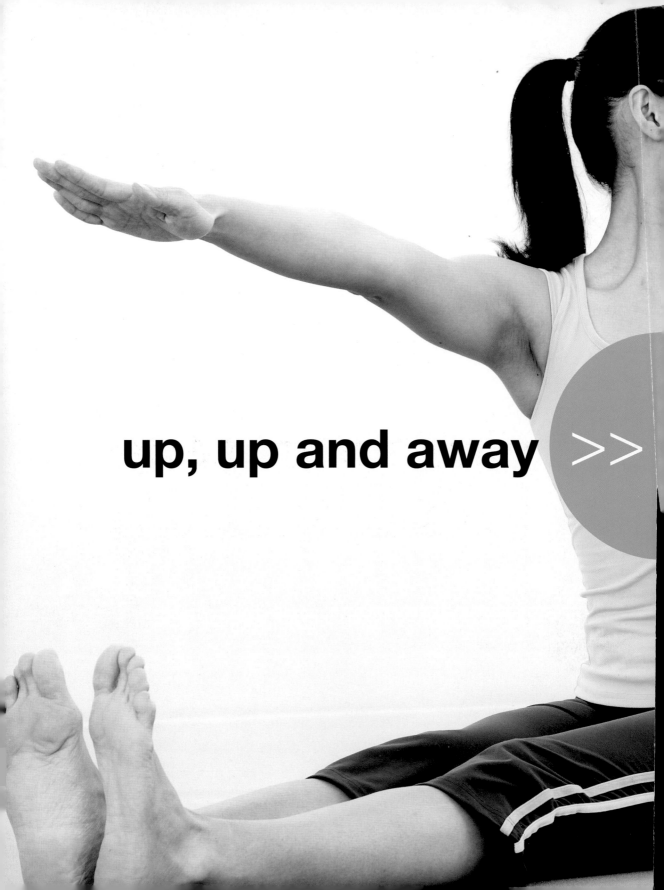

up, up and away >>

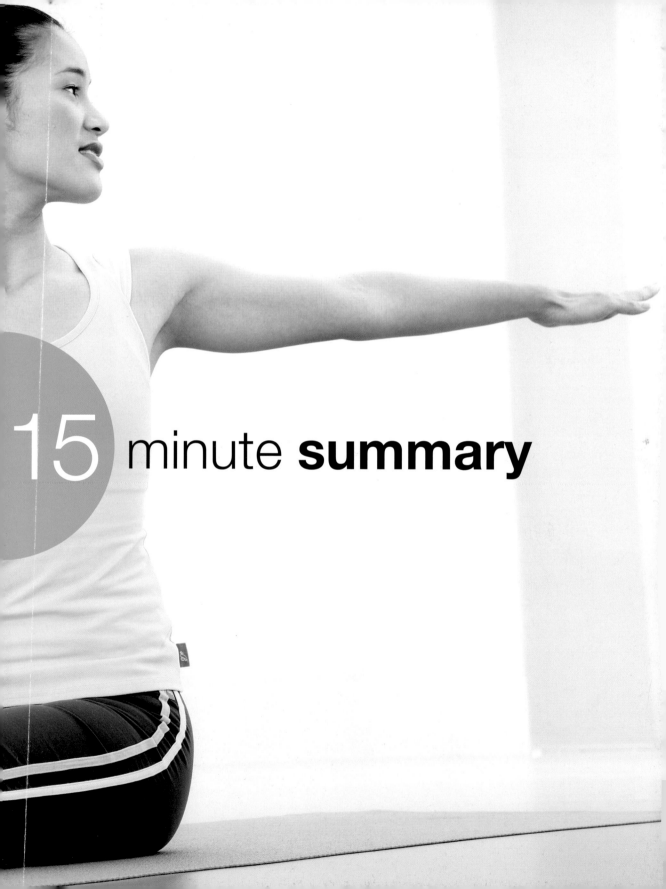

15 minute **summary**

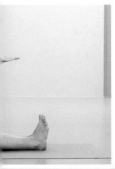

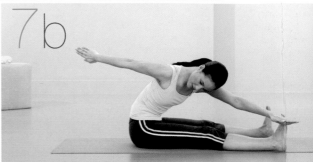

7a

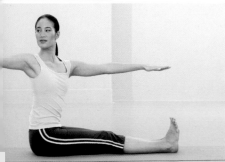

▲ **The Saw**
page 99

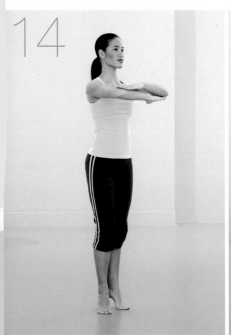

7b

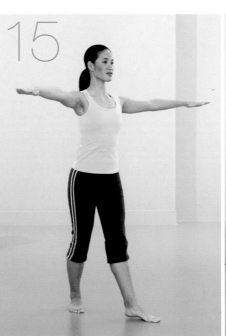

▲ **The Saw** page 99

14

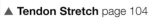

15

16

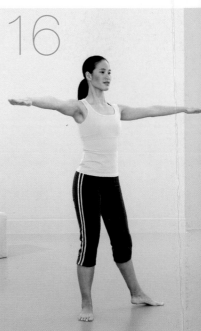

▲ **Tendon Stretch** page 104

▲ **Front Splits** page 105

▲ **Side Splits** page 105

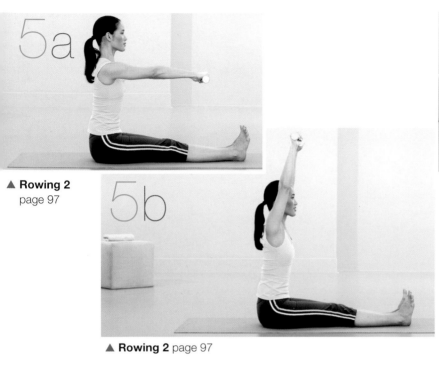

▲ **Rowing 2**
page 97

▲ **Rowing 2** page 97

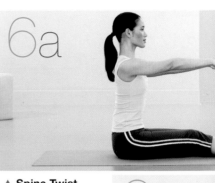

▲ **Spine Twist**
page 98

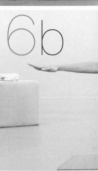

▲ **Spine Twist** page

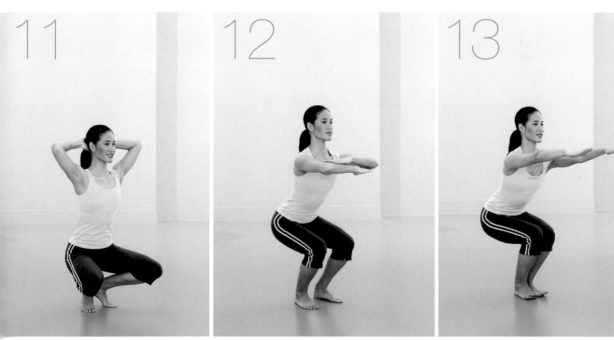

▲ **Footwork 1** page 103

▲ **Footwork 2** page 103

▲ **Footwork 3** page 104

>> **up, up and away** extras

Consider the pace of your everyday life. Do you ever have time truly to prepare for a movement, a reach or a shift of your weight? Not likely. Life happens fast. The ideal exercise routine will prepare you for that speed. Use this routine to prepare for your normal day.

>> **Checklist**

As you work through this programme, be sure not to limit your attention to one area of the body. All of your muscles should work.

• Did you focus on your posture for the whole programme?

• Have you established the feeling of making space between your vertebrae to elongate your spine?

• Can you feel the level of work required in the waistline, and the fatigue it can cause to sit up tall?

• Were you able to keep your inner thighs drawn together and the legs zipped up during the Hundred?

• For the Rowing 1 exercise, the torso is challenged to remain vertical while the arms sweep up and down. Did you manage to initiate the movement from your core to keep your body stable?

• Opening the back arm during the Spine Twist is fairly simple, but turning the whole opposite side of the rib cage to the front is tough. Were you able to spiral around your own spine, lifting taller throughout the torso the whole time?

• At the most intense portion of the Thigh Stretch, where your body is hinged backwards, were you able to tighten your buttocks to create even more stretch in the front of the thighs?

• Timing is everything in the Footwork series. Rather than rushing your body through moves, slowing down slightly will increase the work to your muscles and have a greater benefit.

>> Modify/Adjust

Adding weights to your programme can be a challenge. Practise the exercises without the weights before adding them.

• Soften the knees or sit cross-legged for any seated exercises that cause strain in straight-legged positions.

• Reduce the depth of the knee bends for Footwork 1, 2 and 3.

• Place a cushion under you to protect your knees when kneeling.

• Take your hands across your chest or behind your head as you perform the Spine Twist, to reduce the range.

>> Challenge

Remember, if the exercise doesn't seem challenging, you aren't working hard enough. Review the details and try again.

• Remember, continuously feel the top of your head growing higher up during Rowing 1 and 2.

• Learn to stretch a bit deeper in the Saw – coming up only after you've gone as far as possible.

• Train yourself to work the inner thighs tirelessly whenever seated with the legs together, as in Rowing 1 and 2.

• Try to exaggerate the opposition in twisting or rotary movements.

>> Trainer tips

Be aware that your centre of gravity and balance will change as you rise up through different positions.

• Our bodies follow a developmental sequence from birth to childhood, moving from lying to sitting, kneeling and, finally, standing. This programme takes you through that sequence but gives you the opportunity to check your symmetry.

• When performing the Footwork series, the rising up with control is the hardest movement. Rather than try to get up away from the floor, think of boring a hole into the floor with your feet. The harder you push down, the more the floor will push up against you.

• The Front and Side Splits mirror with the limbs what's going on internally. Envisage your muscles pulling inwards and upwards as the legs pull together.

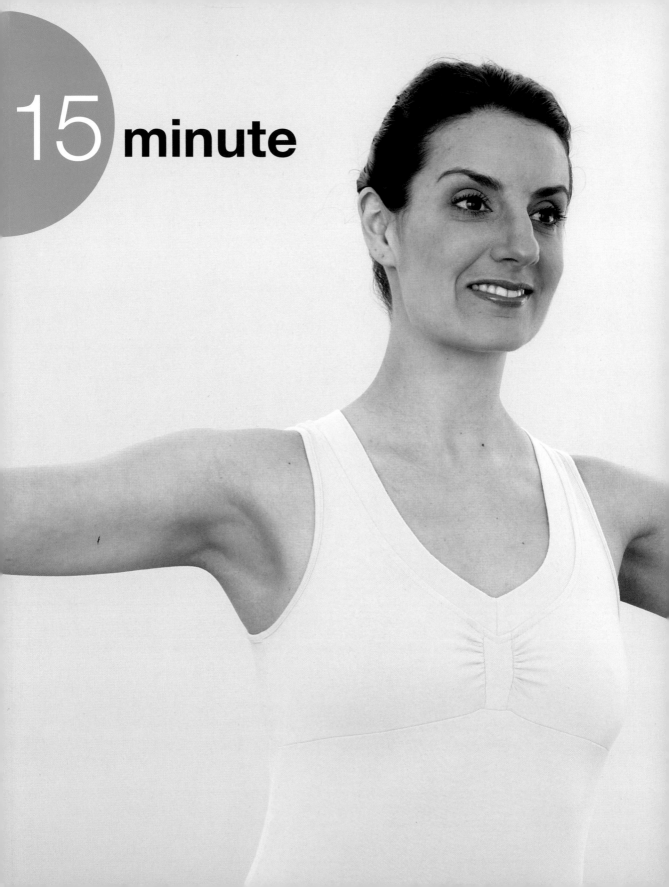

15 minute

Focus on consistency
Activate proper body mechanics
Learn the story of Pilates

beyond the
workout >>

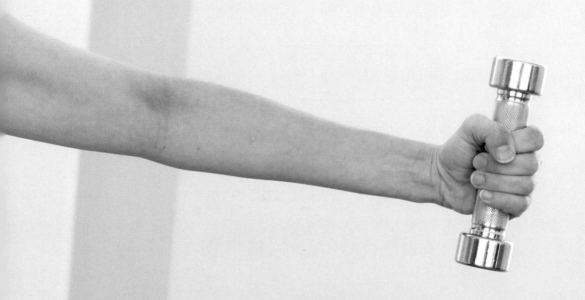

>> **workout** schedule

Everyday Pilates is meant to be accessible, attainable and convenient. Whether it's 15 minutes three times a week or 45 minutes every day to devote to your daily fitness, *Everyday Pilates* can be structured to suit your schedule. Below are three programmes to start you off.

If you only have 15 minutes a day three times a week, simply rotate the four programmes, choosing a different one each day until you've cycled through all four and are ready to begin again. If you can squeeze in between 15 and 30 minutes per day, the Day by Day workout should be done on alternating days three days per week to emphasize and develop the core of the body. On Tuesdays and Thursdays you will get to test how well you can integrate the main principles and positions in the other three programmes in an extended 30-minute workout. If you can manage 30 to 45 minutes a day, I recommend performing the Day by Day workout every day and following up with alternating programmes, choosing one day as your longest workout day.

>> **pilates** workout planner

	Available time 15 minutes, 3 times a week	15–30 minutes a day	30–45 minutes a day
Monday	Day by Day (week 1) Up, Up and Away (week 2) From the Bottom Up (week 3)	Day by Day	Day by Day From the Top Down
Tuesday		Up, Up and Away From the Top Down	Day by Day Up, Up and Away
Wednesday	From the Top Down (week 1) Day by Day (week 2) Up, Up and Away (week 3)	Day by Day	Day by Day From the Bottom Up From the Top Down
Thursday		From the Bottom Up Up, Up and Away	Day by Day Up, Up and Away
Friday	From the Bottom Up (week 1) From the Top Down (week 2) Day by Day (week 3)	Day by Day	Day by Day From the Bottom Up

Built-in flexibility

There is a high degree of flexibility in this series. You can decide to do one programme each day or all four if you choose. In the beginning, it is always wise to ease in slowly, limiting your day to one or two programmes. After two or three weeks, you can attempt a longer routine.

To help keep you on track, ensure that you plan actively for your workout. I recommend that you make a note of it in your diary so that it is given just as much importance as all your other obligations. Always remember that your health and wellness should take centre stage in your everyday life.

If there are days you just can't get to your workout, read about it, or watch the DVD. Either way, studying a physical method without engaging has an astounding benefit. You could actually improve your form, elevate your technique and refine your practice, even without performing the workout. This phenomenon is known as physiological empathy and although it won't build muscle mass or shrink your waist, you can learn and improve significantly by keen observation alone.

Take time to learn about your workout. Simply looking at images and reading about the exercises you do will actually help you improve your practice significantly.

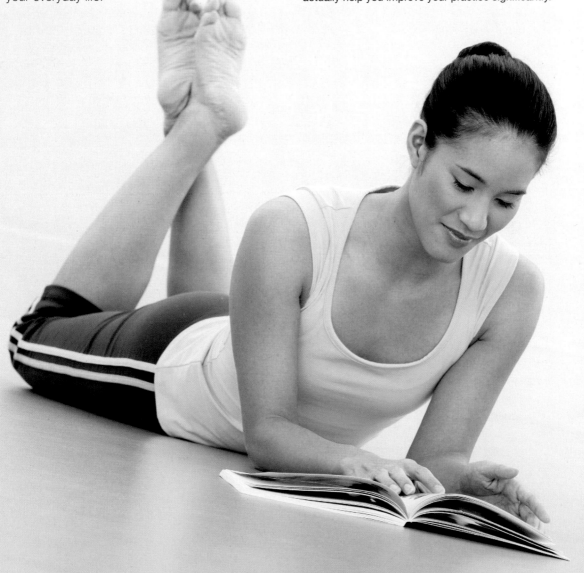

>> **after** the workout

When I attend fitness events I am always amused by a particular phenomenon. After their workouts and at the first opportunity, students revert quickly to their poor posture and slink out of the room with stooped shoulders, sunken chests and protruding midsections. Not so with Pilates.

In your *Everyday Pilates* routines you have been required to build stamina in your postural muscles. The muscles surrounding your spine and running alongside it from your tail to your head have been called upon to perform throughout. Sadly for this particular group of muscles, unless you are lying on your back, they don't get to rest. By working on these postural muscles you are in a better position to employ body mechanics after your workout. When they count the most!

This doesn't mean that poor body mechanics won't resurface occasionally. I am sympathetic to the pull of bad habits. I personally descend from poor posture lineage. For instance, something terrible happens when your body assumes a seated position. All muscle activity arrests. To combat this state of muscle inertia, be sure to leave your chair at regular intervals. At minimum, stand up and reach overhead, stretching your body. Sustained inactivity is unnatural and damaging. When a hospital patient is bedridden, it takes only 12 hours of immobility for bedsores to begin to form. Movement and blood flow are vital to life.

If you are working out and then returning to work, take advantage of the jolt of energy you get immediately after your workout. Rather than revert to a sedentary role, try to keep moving as long as possible. If you commute after your workout, stand for some portion of the trip so your muscles have time to adjust. If you must sit, take the opportunity to work on your sitting posture. Try to keep the chest lifted and the abdominals supported.

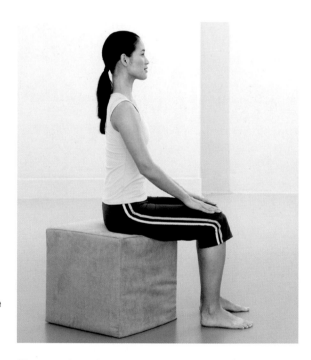

Sit up straight! Once you return to your normal activities, remember to maintain your spinal alignment. Good sitting posture will improve your internal organ function and increase your energy levels.

Stretching

Stretching is good for the body, but never before your workout. Cutting-edge research shows that this is detrimental! Your strength is dramatically reduced as your muscles simply shut off in response. This is not to say you shouldn't stretch. By all means, do. But do so after your workout when your stretching will have the most benefit.

There is always one person in my class stretching away in a straddle position, bobbing up and down trying to get a deeper stretch. Nothing could be less effective. This 'ballistic stretching' actually causes your muscles to contract even tighter. Only by sustained static stretching, that is, holding the stretch completely still and relaxing into it, will you become more flexible. This is the only method of increasing tissue extensibility. If you don't have time to stretch after your workout, do some simple stretches after your shower when your muscles are sufficiently heated.

Soreness

As with any effective training regimen, some soreness is normal. It is caused by micro-tears in the muscle fibre but the good news is that, as the muscle rebuilds, it reshapes into a toned, sculpted and slightly larger version of its former self.

Pilates soreness often occurs two days after a workout and not the very next day. To help alleviate it, make sure to hydrate before you start your workout. On days that you do feel muscle aches, the best remedy is movement. It sounds unlikely, I know. Most people think that you should rest if you feel sore, but by flushing blood through the painful areas you are restoring balance to your system and quickening your healing process. Whenever possible you should perform a few Pilates moves on days that you feel the most sore.

Stretch it out! Stretching should be done only after your workout – never before. This simple hamstring stretch can be done anywhere you can prop up your foot. Simply keep your hips square and your chest lifted. Place your hands on your thigh and gently lean into the stretch.

>> **motivation** tools

Exercise will help you get through your daily life, but life offers you cues to motivate your exercise. If you want to go higher, faster, better, exercise will help you. Mr Pilates understood that motivation is cumulative. He said begin with just 10 minutes a day. That small start can have far-reaching effects.

One of my favourite Pilates quotes is 'Physical fitness can neither be obtained through outright purchase nor wishful thinking.' Overcoming the psychological barriers to exercise can be daunting. Here are a few alternative thoughts to ignite your exercise impulse:

It takes energy to make energy: You will feel more awake, not more tired, after you exercise.

Exercise only works as hard as you do: If you feel low on energy, work out lightly. You do not have to push yourself to the limit each time you work out. It's all right to take it easy on some days.

A workout isn't work: Think of your fitness regime as a luxury. It's maintenance for sure, but it's not a chore for your body; it's more like dessert!

Staying motivated

Here are a couple of my favourite tips for staying motivated that are culled from my clients and staff members:

Rewards: Do something nice for yourself for every week you complete your regime. For instance, have a manicure or buy tickets for an event.

Reality check: Give yourself a break. Simply performing the exercise is enough. If you don't have the energy to put extra effort into it, it will still be beneficial.

Rhythm: It's taboo in the Pilates world, but if you're sure that music will unleash your inner Pilates super-hero, then go for it. Put on your favourite mix of tunes and get started.

Reinforcement: If you like a certain exercise, do

>> **tips to** help your practice

- **Rhythm counts.** Remember to work out at the rhythm of your heart. As you get better, your workout should get shorter and faster.

- **Live Pilates!** Use your Pilates in everyday life to keep you symmetrical and well aligned; stand on equal footing instead of leaning to one side; sit with your ankles crossed instead of your knees; walk with generous strides, leading with your hips as you go.

- **Make a Pact!** Create a support system with a friend to make sure you keep on track no matter what.

some extra ones during the day. You can also take a moment to show someone else how good you are at it. Positive reinforcement goes a long way towards motiviation.

Buddy up

Studies show that people who work out with a friend work out longer and harder. Plan to do Pilates with someone and then police each other so you don't fall off the wagon. It's infinitely harder to turn down a friend than to cheat yourself. And a bit of competition among friends can also be very inspiring. Finally, try teaching a friend some of the moves you've learned. Teaching is very often a learning process. As you dissect and explain the exercises to someone else, you will be absorbing information for your own body.

Be committed

Experts say it takes 21 days to build a new habit. You won't see a change after one workout, but you will feel it! Commit to 21 days of this. Grab a calendar and count off the days. I expect that by the last few days you won't be counting down any more. You'll be counting up instead – counting the increased number of repetitions you are able to perform, the longer workout you're able to get through and, finally, the hours to go until your next great workout.

Complementary workouts

I suggest swimming, weight-training and yoga to complement Pilates: swimming for its non-impact cardiovascular benefits; weight-training to increase bone density and your metabolic rate; yoga for its quiet and stillness. The caveat here is 'mix it up'. Your body will accommodate to training benefits over time and so it is important to change things around periodically. Whatever other type of training you choose, be certain you incorporate all of your Pilates principles. And remember, the best exercise you can do is the one that you enjoy!

Don't go it alone! Change your exercise routine and take a friend along with you. Instead of going out for a coffee, work out together.

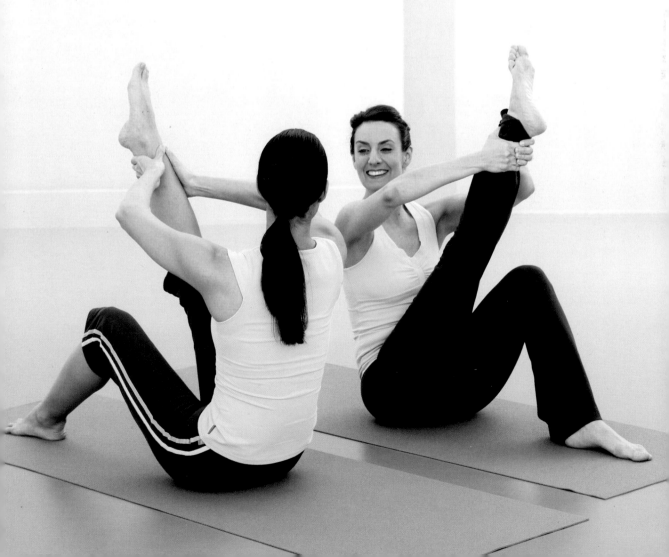

>> **the story** of pilates

Fitness fads come and go. New exercise systems crop up and disappear overnight. Few stand the test of time. Pilates formally established his method in the 1920s and today his system of body conditioning is stronger than ever. Worldwide, some 10 million people practise Pilates. Clearly, Pilates works!

So many versions of the Pilates history exist side by side, it can be hard to weed out the truth. But sometimes it's easier to discern what isn't true, than to look for what is. Here are some of the common myths about Pilates debunked.

• **Pilates is for dancers.** False. Pilates is certainly enjoyed by dancers. But Joseph Pilates did not have a specific audience in mind when he was devising his system.
• **Pilates was a dancer.** No. Joseph Pilates was many things – a diver, gymnast, boxer and acrobat, but he was never a dancer.
• **Pilates is a stretching technique.** No. But every exercise has a lengthening component. A Pilates session can certainly be tailored to address muscular tightness but this is not its sole focus.
• **Pilates requires machines.** Yes. And no. The Pilates Mat work is a total body workout requiring no apparatus. To do the entire Pilates system, one must find a studio with the proper equipment.
• **Pilates is a woman's workout.** Absolutely not. Joseph Pilates did not invent his method for women. In fact, these days men are reclaiming Pilates and there are more male instructors available than ever.

The man

Joseph Pilates was born in 1880 near Dusseldorf in a town called Mönchengladbach. His parents were in the health and fitness fields, his father having been a gymnast and his mother, a naturopath.

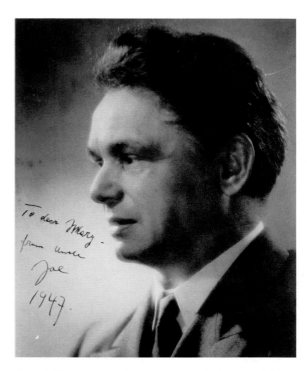

Joseph Pilates was a fitness pioneer who borrowed from ancient disciplines and modern technology to create an entirely new system of body conditioning.

Despite a rocky start as a frail, sickly boy, the young Pilates became passionate about anatomy and movement, and studied yoga as well as Zen and ancient Greek and Roman training regimens. As a result, by the age of 14, he was in extraordinary shape and began to model for anatomy charts.

In reading through the things Joseph Pilates said and his history, it becomes evident that he was indeed a visionary. And that was by no means limited to exercise. One could argue that, with his invention of the Wunda Chair – meant to function as furniture when not used for exercise – he created the first home gym. He also recorded an infomercial of sorts, showing his work and machines to the public. He routinely photographed his clients before and after exercise, to record their dramatic results. Were he alive today, Pilates would be up to date with his marketing strategies. Sadly for him, he did not realize the success of his method in his lifetime.

One of his greatest dreams was to see his method practised in schools worldwide. In the United States today, there is a movement underway and several schools have adopted the system.

The machines

Although Mr Pilates began with his system of floor exercises, he did turn his attention towards the invention of apparatus specifically for his method. His inspiration came from various sources and there is no limit to the tales that surround his creativity. For example, it is often told that Pilates created his Magic Circle (an original thighmaster if you will) from the steel bands of beer kegs. How he came to invent his larger spring-driven equipment was a result of his internship on the Isle of Man during World War I. Pilates was training his captive comrades, many of whom were bedridden. At the

time, hospital beds were constructed with springs so Mr Pilates began to experiment by attaching these springs to the posts of the beds, thereby providing assistance to weakened muscles.

This particular device went through several transformations and is known in the modern Pilates world as the Cadillac or sometimes as the Trapeze Table. In addition, Pilates created a wooden frame with a sliding carriage and variable springs that out-performed his other inventions in terms of variety and accessibility. He labelled this apparatus the Universal Reformer. The Universal Reformer is by far the most commonly used apparatus today and can be found in most, if not all, dedicated Pilates studios around the world.

By the time of his death in 1967, Mr Pilates had created several dozen distinct apparatuses to accompany his tremendous library of exercises.

The method

Today, Pilates is everywhere – in people's homes, on TV and in the gyms. The method is available in some form or other at fitness facilities worldwide. There are fusions, hybrids and cross-training models, all of which are based either fully or in part on the Pilates method.

The Pilates tradition is being passed on to myriad teachers via the five remaining students of Joseph Pilates himself. These master teachers have dedicated their lives to teaching and have passed on their versions, thereby continuing the evolution of the work. Yet, as the method grows, it will become increasingly important to preserve the original work so that the material retains integrity.

What Pilates was or is becoming is less important than what Pilates is to you today. If you experience Pilates as I do, as a comprehensive workout, which delivers the strength, stability and mobility necessary for overall health, then there is simply no reason not to do it.

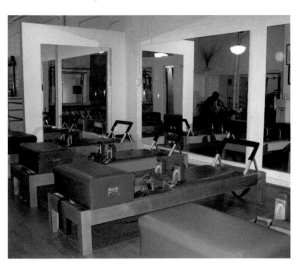

Shown in a studio setting, a row of Universal Reformers, as they are made today. It is the most commonly used Pilates apparatus worldwide.

useful resources

The Pilates method has grown tremendously in recent years and, as a result, hundreds of products are now available to the consumer. Use discretion when choosing Pilates products and be sure to verify the company's credibility and experience with the method. I have listed some reliable sources for all things Pilates-related below.

Finding a Pilates class

Pilates.co.uk
www.pilates.co.uk
A comprehensive website dedicated to the Pilates method, with links to a directory to help you find your nearest Pilates studio or class where you can practice Pilates under the guidance of qualified instructors.

The PILATESfoundation® UK
www.pilatesfoundation.com
The only not-for-profit professional Pilates organization in the UK dedicated to ensuring the highest standards of certification training, continuing education and code of conduct. Has a useful website that is designed to help you find out information about Pilates teachers in your area, as well as supplying information on all aspects of Pilates.

Other books by Alycea Ungaro

Pilates: Body in Motion
(Dorling Kindersley, 2002)
The original resource for the complete Mat repertoire including leveled workouts for beginner, intermediate and advanced exercisers.

The Pilates Promise
(Dorling Kindersley, 2004)
Joseph Pilates made a guarantee that he could give you a whole new body in 30 sessions. Alycea tests his promise with three different women and charts their progress and amazing results.

Pilates Body in Motion Flashcards
(Dorling Kindersley, 2007)
Based on the book, these flashcards are designed for easy portability. Take your favorite exercises with you.

Portable Pilates™ (Pilates Center of New York, 2000)
With user-friendly illustrations, spiral binding and a 38-minute audio workout on CD, this Pilates set is a great primer to take on your travels.

Books by Joseph Pilates

Return to Life through Contrology
(Bodymind Publishing Inc.,1998)
Learn the classic Mat exercises as demonstrated by Joseph Pilates. The complete original Mat work is presented in this historic text.

Your Health
(Presentation Dynamics, 1998)
With recommendations ranging from dry-brushing to proper breathing, this is Mr. Pilates' essay on total wellness.

Audio downloads

Exercise should go where you do. The internet now offers a host of options for accessible exercise.

www.iAmplify.com

Bringing together fitness and lifestyles, iAmplify offers material you can simply load directly onto your desktop, mp3, or iPod for instant accessibility. Log on for live recorded workouts with Alycea.

www.Podfitness.com

Bringing together the top fitness trainers in a variety of disciplines, Podfitness offers you the ability to upload workouts designed by your favorite trainer. Alycea works together with Podfitness to develop Pilates programmes suitable for all levels.

www.realpilatesnyc.com

Alycea Ungaro's free downloads and Pilates printables

Pilates blog

If you have exercise questions specific to Pilates or just want to read what others have to say, a blog is a great source for a variety of information.

PilateSpeak

This blog provides a forum for Pilates professionals and students alike. All questions are answered personally by Alycea.

Equipment

If you are ready to move on to the next level in your Pilates training and invest in some equipment for your home, try the following manufacturers.

Gaiam

www.gaiam.co.uk
Sells equipment for home practise and clothing.

Yoga Mad

www.yogamad.com
Sells mats, weights, small pieces of equipment and clothing.

sweatyBetty

www.sweatyBetty.com
Founded in 1998 by Tamara Hill-Norton, sweatyBetty sells gorgeous clothing for active and not so active women in boutiques nationwide and online.

Pilates periodicals

Although there are dozens of fitness magazines, Pilates has relatively few references devoted to the craft.

Pilates Fitness Journal

www.pilatesfitnessjournal.com
Online monthly Pilates magazine.

Pilates Style Magazine

www.pilatesstyle.com
An American publication available to overseas subscribers.

Pilates for special populations

The Complete Book of Pilates for Men, Daniel Lyon Jr. (Regan Books, 2005)
Promises quick and long-term results to any man who seeks optimal fitness and a competitive edge in all aspects of his life.
Post-Pregnancy Pilates, Karrie Adamany (Avery, 2005)
A guide to heal and reshape a new mother's body. How Pilates can change your body after birth.

For Pilates professionals

Body Control Pilates

www.bodycontrol.co.uk
UK distributor for the Peak Pilates range of Pilates studio equipment from Colorado, USA.

Pilates Institute

www.pilates-institute.com
Established in the UK in 1999, the Pilates Institute is the largest Pilates teacher training company in the UK. The Pilates Institute Method and teacher training programmes are taught throughout the UK and in over 25 countries worldwide.

Pilates Pro

www.pilates-pro.com
Pilates Pro is an online magazine for all Pilates professionals. It provides the industry with access to vital information, tools, services and opportunities that promote community and provide teaching and business solutions.

Stott Pilates®

www.stott-pilates.co.uk
Canadian company that sells Pilates studio equipment. Also provides Pilates instructor training.

index

A

abdominal muscles 16, 40, 41
  Abdominal Curls 23, 40
  Abs Wake-up 22
  breathing 16
  scoop 17, 40
  The Teaser 78, 89
alignment 17, 113
ankle weights 89
arms: Arm Circles 81
  Baby Circles 53, 65
  The Boxing 50
  The Bug 51
  Chest Expansion 101
  Front Curls 46, 64
  The Hug 79
  The Hundred 95, 112
  Lotus 100
  Lunges 54, 64, 65
  The Mermaid 80
  Push-ups 56, 65
  Rowing 96–7, 112
  Salutes 49, 64
  The Saw 99, 113
  Side Bend 55, 64
  Side Curls 47, 64
  triceps 52
  Zip-ups 48, 64

B

Baby Circles 44, 53, 65
back see spine
balance 15
Ball, Rolling like a 33, 40, 41
Beats on Stomach 77, 88
Bicycle Side Kicks 76
body parts 13
The Boxing 50
breathing 15, 16
  the breathing exercise 40
  focusing 65
The Bug 51

buttocks 17
  Pilates stance 68, 70

C

centring 14
Chest Expansion 92, 101
Child's Pose 32
circles: Arm Circles 81
  Baby Circles 44, 53, 65
  Side Kicks 74, 88
  Single Leg Circles 26, 40, 41
clothing 10
concentration 14
connectivity 41
control 14, 15
core stability 14, 64
counter-movements 41
curls: Abdominal Curls 23, 40
  Front Curls 46, 64
  Side Curls 47, 64

D

day by day programme 19–41
Double-leg Stretch 29, 41

E

energy 120
equipment 10

F

feet 17
finishing moves 20, 68
flow of movement 15
footwear 10
footwork 92, 103–4, 112, 113
'frame', working within 17, 64
friends, working with 120–1
Front Curls 46, 64
Front Side Kicks 72, 88
Front Splits 105, 113

H

hamstrings, standing exercises 44
hand weights 10, 44, 65
head, crown of 92
The Hug 79
The Hundred 24, 40, 95, 112

I

Inner-thigh Lifts 75
integration 15
internal resistance 17, 64

J

joints, safety 65

L

'leaning into the wind' 44, 64
legs: alignment 17, 64
  Bbeats on Stomach 77, 88
  Double-leg Stretch 29, 41
  footwork 92, 103–4, 112, 113
  Pilates stance 70, 88
  Push-ups 56, 65
  Side Kicks 71–6, 88, 89
  Single-leg Circles 26, 40, 41
  Single-leg Stretch 28, 41
  standing exercises 44
  Tendon Stretch 104
  Thigh Stretch 92, 102, 112
Lotus 100
lower-body series 66–89
  Arm Circles 81
  Beats on Stomach 77
  The Hhug 79
  The Mermaid 80
  Pilates stance 70
  Side Kicks Bicycle 76
  Side Kicks Circles 74, 88
  Side Kicks Front 72
  Side Kicks Inner-thigh Lifts 75
  Side Kicks Preparation 71
  Side Kicks Up and Down 73

The Teaser 78
Lunges 54, 64, 65

M

mats 10
The Mermaid 68, 69, 80, 89
'mind–body' connection 12
motivation 120–1
moves: connectivity 41
counter-movements 41
finishing 20, 68
flow of movement 15
starting 20, 68
transitioning 20–1, 44, 68, 92
muscles: increasing resistance 41
postural muscles 118
soreness 119
starting moves 68
stretching 118–19

N

neck: alignment 16, 92
Neck Press 94
Neck Roll 31

O

opposition 17, 88

P

pelvis: Pelvic Lift 32, 40
Rolling Like a Ball 33, 40, 41
Pilates, Joseph 12, 15, 122–3
Pilates stance 17, 68, 70, 88, 89
planning workout 116–17
postural muscles 118
powerhouse 16–17
precision 14, 15
principles of Pilates 14–15, 16–17
Push-ups 44, 56, 65

R

repetitions 12, 121, 65
resistance 17
increasing 41
internal 17, 64

rolling: preparation 27, 40
The Roll-Down 25
Rolling Like a Ball 33, 40, 41
Rowing 96–7, 112, 113

S

safety 11
Salutes 49, 64
The Saw 99, 113
scoop 17, 40
self-awareness 12
shoes 10
Shoulder Roll 94
Side Bend 44, 55, 64
Side Curls 47, 64
Side Kicks 88, 89
bicycle 76
circles 74, 88
front 72, 88
Inner-thigh Lifts 75
preparation 71
Up and Down 73
Side Splits 105, 113
Single-leg Circles 26, 40, 41
Single-leg Stretch 28, 41
sitting: cross-legged position 89
Pilates stance 68, 70
socks 10
soreness 119
spine: aligning neck 16, 92
alignment 17
elongating 112
Rolling Like a Ball 33, 40, 41
Salutes 49, 64
Spine Stretch Forwards 30, 40
Spine Twist 98, 112, 113
Zip-ups 48, 64
splits 105, 113
stability, core 14, 64
stance 17, 70, 88, 89
initiating 68
standing exercises 44
starting moves 20, 68
strength training 17
stretches 118–19

Double-leg Stretch 29, 41
Single-leg Stretch 28, 41
Spine Stretch Forwards 30, 40
Tendon Stretch 104
Thigh Stretch 92, 102, 112
The Swan 31
swimming 121
symmetry 15, 17

T

The Teaser 78, 89
Tendon Stretch 104
Thigh Stretch 92, 102, 112
transitions 20–1, 41, 44, 68, 92
Triceps 52
twists 113
Spine Twist 98, 112, 113

U

Up and Down Side Kicks 73
Up, Up and Away 91–113
upper-body series 42–65
Baby Circles 53
The Boxing 50
The Bug 51
Front Curls 46
Lunges 54
Push-ups 56
Salutes 49
Side Bend 55
Side Curls 47
Triceps 52
Windmill 57
Zip-ups 48

W, Y, Z

weights 10, 113, 65
ankle weights 89
hand-weight series 44, 65
increasing 65
weight-training 121
Windmill 57
workout schedule 116–17
yoga 121
Zip-ups 48, 64

acknowledgments

Author's acknowledgments

I was aware during the creation of this project that no task is accomplished alone. I am filled with gratitude for so many people for their constant support, but particularly my mother, Susan Baylis and my husband, Robert Ungaro, both of whom are responsible for any successes I may have achieved. I want also to thank my delicious girls Emma and Estelle, who tolerated weeks of a busy mum in the name of this project.

Thanks go to the inimitable publicists of D2 Publicity for making sure the world knows about us and Laurie Liss @ Sterling Lord Literistic for her agenting prowess. I also thank the beauty squad: Anton Thompson and Mary Schook, as well as Kent Mancini, Victoria Barnes and Roisin Donaghy.

At DK I wish to thank Mary-Clare Jerram, Miranda Harvey, Penny Warren and Hilary Mandleberg, who understood when the chips were down that long pants were the key to happiness. Shout outs go to the phenomenal team at Alycea Ungaro's Real Pilates, including the instructors who lend me their words and inspiration every day. Deep and profound appreciation goes out to the administrative team that runs my business and hence my life while I sequester myself to write and create. They are: Casey Kern (boss of everything), Jan Phillips (ruler of all) and Shelley Hardin (graphics goddess).

I am incredibly thankful to Joel Mishcon for his vision and direction and, of course, to Charlie Arnaldo, who lent her form, eye and talent to this project and ultimately 'made it happen'.

Special thanks to Amara Leyton for lending me her mum, Melody, while I go to work every day and also to Benjamin and Adeline Teolis for offering their mother, Loren, for hours of phone consultation.

Publisher's acknowledgments

Dorling Kindersley thanks photographer Ruth Jenkinson and her assistants, James McNaught and Vic Churchill; sweatyBetty for the loan of the exercise clothing; Viv Riley at Touch Studios; the models Rhona Crewe and Sam Johannesson; Roisin Donaghy and Victoria Barnes for the hair and makeup; YogaMatters for supplying the mat.

Thanks also to Mary Pilates, niece of Joseph Pilates, for her generosity in supplying the photograph of Mr Pilates on page 122 and to Alycea Ungaro's Real Pilates for the photograph of the Pilates studio on page 123.

about Alycea Ungaro

Alycea Ungaro, PT, is the owner of Alycea Ungaro's Real Pilates in New York City and the author of several best-selling Pilates titles including *Portable Pilates*™, *Pilates: Body in Motion* and *The Pilates Promise*, some of which are available in 17 languages worldwide. Alycea's personal mission is to make Pilates available to everyone regardless of age, fitness level, or geographic location. To that end, Alycea has created Pilates products in every possible medium. She presents seminars and workshops nationally and also serves on the advisory board of *Fitness Magazine*. Alycea is a featured personality on podfitness.com and iamplify.com, where you can download her signature workouts to your desktop or iPod. She lives in New York City with her family. To learn more about Alycea or Alycea Ungaro's Real Pilates, visit www.realpilatesnyc.com